ADHD/Hyperactivity:
A CONSUMER'S GUIDE

For
Parents
and
Teachers

To Stan —
Read + enjoy!
Thanks for listening!
Michael Gordon

Michael Gordon, Ph.D.

Professor of Psychiatry
Director, Attention Deficit Hyperactivity Disorders Clinic
SUNY Health Science Center at Syracuse

GSI Publications
PO Box 746 • DeWitt, NY 13214
(315) 446-4849

GSI Publications
PO Box 746
DeWitt, NY 13214
(315) 446-4849

This publication is designed to provide accurate and authoritative information in regard to the subject matter covered. It is sold with the
understanding that the publisher is not engaged in rendering legal,
psychological, or other professional services. If legal, psychological
service or other expert assistance is required, the services of a competent professional person should be sought.

ISBN 0-9627701-0-8

Library of Congress Catalog Card Number 90-084127

Acknowledgments

While only one name is listed as author, you will find that this book uses the voice of "We" instead of "I" throughout the text. This is not simply a stylistic vehicle or an early sign of multiple personality disorder. Instead, it reflects my full awareness of the extent to which so many colleagues have, in one way or another, contributed to this work. Using "We" is my acknowledgment of their talents and contributions. It also captures the close-knit collaboration among the faculty, staff, and trainees involved in our Attention Deficit Hyperactivity Disorders Clinic.

Several individuals were especially helpful in reviewing this manuscript. Dr. Russell Barkley, always an inspiration and support, contributed his vast expertise, as did Dr. Martin Irwin, Head of the Division of Child and Adolescent Psychiatry in my department. Ms. Barbara Mettelman, Coordinator of our Clinic, provided technical savvy and a multitude of fine suggestions, not to mention her usual loyalty and encouragement. Stylistic niceties were masterfully attended to by Dr. Ruth Burton, a wonderful editor and even better friend. My wife, Dr. Wendy Gordon, not only made valuable contributions to the manuscript, but also refrained from committing justifiable homicide while I was busy with this project. I very much appreciate the efforts of Mrs. Dianne Graves and Mrs. JoAnne C. Baker, mothers of ADHD children, whose input was extremely useful. I also want to thank Drs. Ernest M. Post, Harvey C. Parker, F. Daniel McClure, and Deborah DiNiro as well as Robert C. Paltz, Esq. for their unflagging encouragement and sage counsel.

If you like the look of this book, it's because of the graphic wizardry of Ms. Janet Junco. Her willingness to put up with my endless questions and intrusions marks her as a prime candidate for sainthood. I also appreciate the keen eyes of Ms. Lisa MacLachlan and Ms. Mary McCargar, who proofread the various drafts and galleys.

The real hidden authors of this book are the hundreds of parents, children and teachers I've worked with over the years. It's one thing to read books and journal articles about ADHD/Hyperactivity, but quite another to hear the insights and experiences of all those involved on a daily basis with this vexing problem. I hope that you find your thoughts and concerns faithfully woven into these pages.

Michael Gordon, Ph.D.
Syracuse, NY
7/22/90

To Wendy and the Blues Brothers
(a.k.a. Alexander and Joshua)

Contents

Preface

Parents of hyperactive children or of youngsters suspected of being hyperactive confront a barrage of confusing information about how best to proceed with evaluation and treatment. So many different professionals are involved in the management of this problem and so many fad theories and quick-cures are offered that parents often feel at a loss to know how best to help their children. Most parents will consult four or five different practitioners before receiving a meaningful diagnosis and a reasonable treatment program. Unfortunately, thousands of dollars and valuable time are lost as parents wend their way through a maze of services.

This book is intended as a consumer's guide for those seeking resources for the hyperactive or "maybe" hyperactive child. We prepared this material by asking ourselves, "What do all those research studies about hyperactivity really have to say of import to parents and teachers of these children?" To be useful, we will not present a traditional recounting of the history of hyperactivity research or an academic discussion of theories. Nor are we looking to offer a comprehensive review of the field, because much of this material is already available (and listed in the "Resources" section at the end of this book). Instead, we will discuss 30 "Principles" which we feel can guide all of us working with these children.

Our hope is that your understanding of these Principles will make you a more sophisticated consumer of professional services and a more effective advocate for your child. At the very least, we want to help you avoid some of the most serious pitfalls that can be so costly in terms of money, effort and disappointment. While many of the points we will be making would find general agreement among our colleagues, several clearly reflect our own vigorous biases. We'll do our best to indicate which principles are most controversial.

Much of the material you will be reading stems from fifteen years of research and clinical practice involving children referred because of overactivity, impulsiveness, and inattention. Our Attention Deficit Hyperactivity Disorders Clinic has evaluated more than 500 children over the past five years and we have had extensive contact with parent support groups across the country. The motivation to write this book stems from our sense of a deep need for accurate information that is presented in a format parents find down-to-earth and practical.

The underlying theme of this book is that evaluation and treatment for ADHD/Hyperactivity should proceed in a careful and systematic fashion. Even at the risk of sounding overly-cautious or skeptical, we constantly warn of pitfalls and panaceas. As you will read, there are neither magical tests nor miracle remedies for this complex disorder. But you will also learn about reasonable approaches to evaluation and treatment.

We understand that you may already have gone through an evaluation and do indeed have a hyperactive child. Our early remarks regarding appropriate diagnosis are not intended to cast doubt upon decisions already made. For the benefit of those who are unsure whether or not their child is hyperactive and to illustrate where we as professionals stand in regard to conceptualizing this disorder, we will spend considerable time on diagnostic issues.

While we address many of our remarks directly to parents, we hope that teachers will find the information useful in better understanding their hyperactive students and perhaps in gaining perspective on the child's life beyond the classroom. We have also included considerable material on educational issues and specific techniques for effective classroom management. In fact, you will find that we shift from "talking" to parents to addressing teachers during several sections devoted entirely to educational issues.

You will notice that we use the terms "ADHD" and "Hyperactivity" interchangeably. "ADHD" stands for Attention Deficit Hyperactivity Disorder and is the official term sanctioned by the American Psychiatric Association. Physicians and mental health workers refer to hyperactive children as having an Attention Deficit Hyperactivity Disorder (or ADHD). Just to confuse us all a bit further, "ADHD" recently replaced "ADD" (Attention Deficit Disorder) as the official label. You will still see books and articles using "ADD" instead of "ADHD," but they are referring essentially to the same problem.

We researchers have had no difficulty coming up with a variety of labels to describe the same set of problem behaviors. At one point several years ago the government had a list of no less than 98 terms, including such labels as minimal brain dysfunction, minimal cerebral dysfunction, hyperkinesis, and overactivity disorder. Even though the term "Hyperactivity" is no longer official, we still use it occasionally because it is so common. Actually, whenever possible we dodge the whole issue of which term is best and call the disorder "ADHD/Hyperactivity."

Incidentally, the shift away from terms focusing on activity level to those highlighting attention deficits reflects an overall change in our thinking which has moved away from looking primarily at the sheer quantity of behavior toward concentrating on the quality of the child's behavior. What sets hyperactive children apart is that their behavior tends to be poorly organized and planned. A central problem concerns the child's inability to pay attention and to sustain effort.

Now let's turn to the first of our guiding principles for comprehensive evaluation and treatment.

PRINCIPLE 1

Seek the Best in Evaluation Before You Seek the Best in Treatment

You will read in this book about the many complexities that are inherent in properly understanding and evaluating ADHD/Hyperactivity in children. Many children who are **not** truly hyperactive exhibit some or many of the behaviors associated with the disorder. Even children who fit criteria for ADHD represent not one uniform group, but a variety of subgroups, each requiring different treatment programs. We will be covering these issues carefully in later sections. The point we want to drive home first is that it is, in our opinion, an error to skip lightly over evaluation and run headlong into treatment.

You can't blame anyone for wanting to leap right to the "cure." Evaluations tend to be time-consuming and costly and, unfortunately, are often done in such a way that they do not have much meaning for treatment. However, evaluations can be conducted in a highly relevant and cost-effective fashion. We will be reviewing what to look for in a clinician and an evaluation.

The appeal of a quick cure is intense for all of us, because this is a difficult problem which taxes families terribly. There is a high level of marital discord in families of hyperactive children — discord that is often related to the stress of managing a highly unmanageable child. Mothers of hyperactive children tend to experience a depression which is related, at least in part, to the despair inherent in trying to deal with a child who seems designed to make a parent feel inept, impotent, rageful and guilty. The desire of parents to bypass the more demanding process of careful evaluation and comprehensive treatment is thus wholly understandable.

Not only parents but also clinicians find this a frustrating disorder with which to deal. While we professionals have come a long way in arriving at a consensus about how to evaluate children who are referred to us for hyperactivity, criteria are still quite subjective and guidelines tend to be vague. Out of frustration, we too often look for easy solutions that can lead our patients down the wrong path.

Finally, in an effort to avoid feeling a sense of responsibility and guilt, many parents and especially educators are, at times, too quick to pin a label of ADHD on a child. Frankly, some schools will call a child ADHD instead of emotionally disturbed because they feel that parents will better accept this more "medical" diagnosis than they will a label that denotes emotional disturbance. At times, children are labeled ADHD/ Hyperactive when their problems stem more directly from poor child rearing practices or problems at home. Again, clinicians and schools find it easier to call the child ADHD than to deal with vexing issues of parental responsibilities. It can also be the case that a child is labeled hyperactive because he or she experiences problems with the educational environment. It is sometimes less troublesome to call the child hyperactive than to deal with his learning style, a teacher's teaching style, or with faults in the curriculum.

The general point is straightforward: successful solutions come from first understanding the nature of the problem itself. Conversely, solutions that are applied before understanding the problem can often miss the mark. Missing the mark in this arena takes on considerable significance. Misdiagnoses can lead to the unnecessary prescription of medications that have known potential side effects. Rushing to treatment can also lead to treating children who either do not need help or require services other than those appropriate for the ADHD/ Hyperactive child.

The need for a comprehensive evaluation stems largely from the fact that there are no clear-cut markers or signs that invariably identify the presence of the disorder. There is no single physical feature, blood test, brain wave indicator or score on any particular psychological measure that a clinician can look at and say, "Ah ha, he's got it!" It would certainly make it easier for us to secure services (not to mention insurance reimbursements) for ADHD children if we could point to an ADHD child's forehead and declare, "There it is, the green telltale mark of ADHD sitting two inches above the right eyebrow" but, alas, this is a condition which calls for a more challenging investigation.

The absence of sure-shot signs of ADHD unfortunately hasn't stopped many a professional from coming up with his or her own trusty test for ADHD. Some will make decisions based on responses to a simple question or two: "Does he sleep quietly through the night or constantly toss and turn?" "Can he sit for TV or Nintendo?" "Will he sit through a meal?" While many ADHD children are restless sleepers or have trouble sitting for TV and meals, just as many bonafide ADHD children sleep relatively motionless and are able to keep still for a TV show or computer game. Again, we have yet to (and most likely will not) uncover a litmus test for ADHD. Like it or not, the evaluation for ADHD resembles more a detective's search for clues than a prospector's declaration of gold in the hills.

PRINCIPLE 2

All That Is Hyper Is Not Hyperactivity

ADHD/Hyperactivity is as popular a disorder as it is hard to define. Unambiguous criteria for evaluating a child as hyperactive have been most elusive because, especially in younger children, the boundaries between normal and abnormal behavior are slender. Even the best behaved child can go through phases where he fits many of the behavioral criteria for hyperactivity. As you will also learn, some children are not obviously overly-active, but nevertheless exhibit significant problems in maintaining attention.

Before explaining concepts that underlie current no-tions about ADHD/Hyperactivity, we first want to illus-trate with actual case histories some of the complexities which confront us when people come to our clinic with the question, "Is my child hyperactive?." Presentation of these cases should give you a feel for the many issues involved when a child is considered as potentially hyper-active. Our intention is not, however, to portray ADHD/ Hyperactivity as an insurmountable problem, nor do we want to convey the notion that most evaluations are mishandled by parents and professionals (although one of the joys inherent in writing about prior cases is that you can pick instances where you look particularly tal-ented and others come across as bumbling at best). Also, as with all the cases presented in this book, many details have been altered to protect confidentiality.

A typical referral to our clinic was made by a local pediatrician who was concerned about eight year old

Tommy Reed. Six months prior to this visit, the boy's parents had told the physician that their son was increasingly difficult for them to control. He was refusing to complete his homework, was always on the move, and constantly argued with his older brother. The parents were earnest in their efforts to help Tommy learn to better control himself. They would try one method or another for a few weeks at a time, always without enduring success. They indicated that Tommy was an affectionate and caring child but one who found it hard to express his emotions freely.

Tommy's school reported that, although popular with peers, he often did not sit in his seat long enough to complete work up to what they thought was his high potential. His papers were poorly organized and messy. He also had a habit of leaving his chair to wander about the room. Unfortunately, Tommy was in a large class of 29 children, several of whom presented the teacher with similar challenges.

As with many parents who come for an evaluation, the Reeds had already sought advice from a variety of professionals who, in turn, offered often conflicting opinions and confusing recommendations. The family's first stop was to their pediatrician. He suggested that Mrs. Reed was overly-concerned about a boy who, in his opinion, was just rambunctious and energetic. The doctor reassured them that Tommy was physically and neurologically healthy, and that he would "grow out" of his current difficulties. He told the Reeds that they should "loosen up" on Tommy and work with the school to cure the boy's lack of motivation.

The Reeds did schedule a meeting with Tommy's teachers and guidance counselor. The consensus of opinion was that Tommy was too distracted by all the social activity of a relatively chaotic classroom and would benefit from less stimulation. In order to minimize distractions, they decided to seat Tommy in a front corner of the room with two dividers to the side and back of his desk. One of the teachers, while agreeing with this approach, told Mrs. Reed that she had just come from a professional workshop and thought that Tommy sounded like children who were described as having an Attention Deficit Hyperactivity Disorder.

Mrs. Reed had heard about hyperactivity from a friend whose son had been diagnosed as such by another pediatrician. While she felt that Tommy was not nearly as problematic as her friend's child, she was concerned by some similarities in their behavior. On the advice of another friend, the Reeds called a local mental health clinic for an evaluation.

This particular agency had a reputation for innovative approaches to managing family problems. After two diagnostic visits during which information was gathered, the case worker told the Reeds that, in his opinion, family problems were contributing to Tommy's difficulties. He felt that Mrs. Reed tended to dominate the family system and did not allow other members to assume their appropriate roles. The case worker also suggested that Mr. Reed was too passive in his involvement in the family. The consequence of this uneven balance of authority in the family was Tommy's oppositional behavior and lack of discipline.

The agency's recommendation was that the Reeds engage in family therapy to correct these maladaptive family patterns. At the same time, the case worker thought that Tommy might be "a little hyperactive" and suggested that they monitor his diet for foods that made him "hyper." He gave the Reeds the name of a local allergist who could assist them in exploring the possibility that food allergies contributed to Tommy's fidgetiness.

The Reeds followed through on both recommendations and came into the mental health clinic for nine appointments, during which a host of family and personal issues were discussed. They also met with the allergist who ran a series of tests and suggested that they put Tommy on a restricted diet which eliminated milk, chocolate and all foods containing sodium nitrite.

Despite these efforts, Tommy's behavior at home and school continued to deteriorate. He found it increasingly difficult to attend to his work. The school became more convinced that Tommy was hyperactive and told the parents that he needed medication to function at a grade-appropriate level. The Reeds, now becoming frustrated and somewhat desperate, returned to the pediatrician so that he could prescribe the medication.

Because the situation had worsened over the six months since he had last examined Tommy, the doctor took the parent and school complaints more seriously and began to consider the possibility that the boy was indeed hyperactive. To his credit, however, he was not comfortable prescribing medication without further documentation of the boy's attention deficits. The physician also made it clear that he was not an expert in this area and would welcome the input of our ADHD/ Hyperactivity Clinic. When Mrs. Reed called us for an appointment she rather pointedly demanded that we, once and for all, tell her whether or not her son was hyperactive.

Was Tommy Reed hyperactive? On its surface, the case initially looked to us like a rather uncomplicated instance of ADHD/Hyperactivity. All the hallmarks were in evidence: a history of academic underachievement, inattention, and fidgetiness despite normal intelligence and the absence of obvious emotional or neurological problems. But before telling you the outcome of this evaluation, we will briefly describe other cases that seemed similarly "open-and-shut."

Ken, a 10 year old boy, was referred for a psychological evaluation by both his school and pediatrician. According to all concerned, Ken was consistently impulsive, disruptive, inattentive, hyperactive and underachieving. Judging from rating scales and case-history information, his behavior met all the accepted criteria for a diagnosis of ADHD/Hyperactivity. The age of onset for his problems was before 5 years 11 months, his symptoms were chronic and pervasive, his IQ was well over 70, and ratings of his behavior by teachers on standardized checklists all suggested severe problems with impulsiveness and sustained attention. His school had demonstrated ample patience with his misbehavior to the extent that they allowed him to run the hallways for five minutes whenever he could no longer contain his energy. At the time of the referral, the school was reaching the end of its capacity to deal with Ken. School officials wanted us to document his hyperactivity so he could be placed on medication and possibly referred to a residential treatment facility.

Donald, age 6, also came to us for an evaluation because his school, an exclusive private facility, could no longer tolerate his behavior. All the teachers and school staff who had contact with Donald described him as being in constant motion. His primary teacher, though loving and patient, was exasperated by his intensity and drive; she was also frustrated by Donald's single-mindedness and persistence. Though admired for his fertile imagination and unusual artistic abilities, Donald was not liked by his classmates because he would tease them and "act weird." Though the parents did not experience these same kinds of problems with Donald at home, the repeated complaints from school led them to seek an evaluation. In fact, the school informed the parents that Donald would not be permitted to return the following year unless his hyperactivity were brought under control.

Finally, there is the case of 11 year old Marianne who was referred to the clinic for monitoring of her medication. Marianne had been diagnosed at the age of 7 as hyperactive because her mother found her unusually difficult to manage. She refused to follow rules and argued with mother about everything. Marianne was very aggressive with her younger sister and demanded everybody's attention. The mother told us that, without the medication, her daughter made life around the house "a living hell."

All the children described above fit common descriptions of the ADHD/Hyperactive youngster. Each one was difficult for adults to manage, tended to do things without first thinking, and experienced some degree of academic and social maladjustment. Are they all ADHD/Hyperactive?

According to generally accepted criteria (which you will read about shortly), Tommy Reed's case certainly seemed most suitable for the diagnosis of ADHD/Hyperactivity. Both parents and teachers complained about his impulsivity and inattentiveness, and there was no evidence of a physical or neurological disease. During the initial appointment, the Reeds recounted Tommy's symptoms and their efforts to secure appropriate services. Because none of their past efforts seemed to help, they were more and more convinced that Tommy was hyperactive. Their responses to a series of behavior problem checklists all suggested that Tommy was indeed hyperactive and inattentive. Materials that had been sent from the school generally supported this diagnosis. One of the teachers, although she thought Tommy was a difficult child to handle, was not convinced he was hyperactive.

As the evaluation progressed, some information developed which began to make us question the validity of labeling Tommy as hyperactive. Unlike many ADHD/ Hyperactive children who are difficult to manage from early in their lives and never seem to outgrow the "terrible two's," Tommy was reportedly an easy-going infant and toddler who was neither unusually active nor hard to control. At preschool and kindergarten he played well and struck the teachers as bright, pleasant and persevering. Academic and behavior problems surfaced only when he entered first grade.

Another unusual feature of the picture was Tommy's successful peer relationships. As you will read, one of the hallmarks of ADHD/Hyperactivity is profound difficulties with peers. Yet Tommy was popular and tended to play well with other children. He received frequent invitations to birthday parties and was considered by parents in the neighborhood to be the "right kind of friend" for their child.

The final tipoff came when Tommy was tested for his ability to sustain attention. His scores generally fell in the Normal range, although he was quite slow to respond to demands of the various tasks. The examiner noticed that Tommy had difficulty understanding the instructions and needed an unusual amount of help in order to comprehend what was required of him. She also noted that Tommy was nervous about his performance on these tests and tried hard to avoid taking them by asking questions and talking about his hobbies.

Because we were suspicious that there was more than met the proverbial eye in Tommy's case, we referred him for a learning disabilities evaluation. We wanted to know if Tommy's difficulty attending was at all related to a specific problem with processing and understanding language.

The ensuing report was quite striking. Although bright and motivated, Tommy was found to experience significant delays in his ability to process language. He had particular problems interpreting material presented to him verbally. The learning disabilities specialist concluded that Tommy suffered from a specific learning disability that precluded him from performing adequately in school and that most likely affected his self-esteem.

Following a series of conferences with the school, Tommy was identified as "Learning Disabled" and received special educational services on a daily basis. The special education teacher was rather ingenious and always supportive in her work with Tommy. In addition to helping him learn to overcome his educational handicap, she worked with him to feel more comfortable in the classroom. As with so many learning disabled youngsters, Tommy had previously coped with frustrations in the classroom by becoming avoidant. He would rather get in trouble for failing to complete his work than to "feel stupid" in his attempts to complete a difficult assignment. A sheet of written work could just as well have been calculus or Greek, and held about as much of his interest. Children are no different than their adult counterparts when it comes to taking the path of least resistance in the face of daunting obstacles, even if that path leads to uncompleted assignments and upset teachers.

Special educational efforts had relatively quick payoffs for Tommy and his parents. Not as frustrated and

anxious about his competence, Tommy was more manageable at home and school. When we contacted the
Reeds a year after their initial clinic appointment, he
was still receiving special services, but no longer was re-
garded by them or the teachers as hyperactive.

With Ken, the boy who needed to run the hallways
"to burn off energy," the story was quite different. Even
though everyone who knew Ken testified to his hyperactivity, we were not convinced. When we screened him
initially for attention deficits, he came across as highly
anxious and fearful. Unlike most children diagnosed as
hyperactive, Ken was concerned about the adequacy of
his performance while working on the various tasks. He
complained that things happened too quickly for him to
respond, and would slap himself in the face when he
missed an item on one of the tests.

Our suspicions were heightened when we learned
that the onset of his hyperactivity at age 5 coincided
with the gunshot murder of his mother. Because his biological father was unavailable (Ken was born out-of-
wedlock), Ken was raised by his maternal grandparents.
The grandparents were devoted to Ken but, because of
their own fears, suspicions and ambivalence about their
custody of him, they seriously limited his contacts with
others. They also engaged in what appeared to be bi-
zarre rituals around the memory of the boy's mother.
Every night they would light dozens of candles around a
shrine of her pictures and personal belongings. Ken was
encouraged to "talk" to her so that she might keep in
communication with him and know how he was faring.

Ken was referred for a complete psychiatric evaluation to explore the possibility that his school behavior
was more accurately a reflection of severe emotional
problems than of hyperactivity, *per se.* The results of

that assessment indicated that Ken suffered from relatively profound psychiatric disturbance. The family history as well as a host of other factors left Ken with intense fears and a dependent, hostile relationship with his grandparents. As he grew older, he found it increasingly difficult to manage his anxieties and anger. He would become so flooded by stress and confusion that he would often have difficulty organizing himself for even the simplest of tasks. Intensive psychotherapy both with Ken as well as with his grandparents was initiated with good results. He was also transferred to a class for emotionally handicapped children so that he could benefit from additional support and guidance.

Donald, the 6 year-old who caused so much upheaval at the private school, was another child who appeared hyperactive but proved otherwise. Although described by his teachers as a "holy terror," Donald behaved with consummate poise and grace in our offices. His verbal and conceptual abilities were highly advanced for a first grader. He also impressed us as a serious, inquisitive and intense child who constantly sought out stimulation and challenge. Based on his behavior in our clinic, we began to doubt that he was hyperactive. Yet at the same time we knew that hyperactive children were notorious for their capacity to behave well in a doctor's office despite a long legacy of misbehavior in other settings.

On tests of attention and self-control (which will also be described in later chapters), Donald performed well above average; he evidenced no obvious difficulties developing strategies for self-control and vigilance. The examiner noted his overly-mature and industrious style of interaction. In fact, Donald complained to him about how bored he was at school and how the teacher kept him from doing "fun" things. What did Donald consider "fun"? It turns out that his favorite academic pursuit was teaching himself Chinese characters in the hope that one day he might travel to the Orient with his father (who was a college professor of languages). Donald was not about to attend to math problems he was able to manage in preschool when the lure of more stimulating material was at hand. When the teacher forbade his "doodling," he could not tolerate the daily tedium and decided to keep himself busy in more provocative and disruptive ways.

Increasingly convinced that Donald did not suffer from ADHD/Hyperactivity, we suggested to his parents that they have him evaluated with the standard battery of intelligence and personality tests. The results of that assessment confirmed some of our hunches about Donald's school problems. The intelligence tests indicated that Donald was an unusually gifted child whose IQ was measured at 148 (most of us have IQ scores somewhere around 100). His reading, spelling, and math achievement scores were all at or above the fourth grade level.

The personality tests painted the picture of a youngster who felt somewhat isolated from others and always more comfortable pursuing his own particular interests. An only child with advanced intellectual abilities, he never developed a sense of ease in his relationships with other children. As with so many gifted children, Donald exhibited a wide gap between his intellectual and his social/ emotional development. We concluded, therefore, that this was an extremely bright, driven boy who most likely was bored by a school situation which met neither his academic nor his emotional needs. We theorized that much of his untoward behavior reflected his poor interpersonal skills and his chafing against an unstimulating environment.

Many children, especially bright and energetic youngsters, will find one way or another of making a situation sufficiently exciting to maintain their interest and involvement — no matter what it takes and how much trouble it causes. Children abhor boredom the way nature abhors a vacuum.

We suggested to Donald's parents that they investigate the options available for gifted children. After a careful search, they enrolled Donald in a program within their school district. This unique setting was designed to provide an enriched academic environment along with sensitivity to the emotional issues that often confront the gifted child. Donald adjusted to this program quickly and, although still considered by peers as "a little weird," he did not engage in the kinds of behaviors that brought him to us for an ADHD/Hyperactivity evaluation. In fact, he was described by the teaching team as one of their most attentive and well-behaved students.

The case of Marianne illustrates another instance in which a child can be mislabeled "hyperactive" as a result of an incomplete evaluation of the symptoms. This attractive 11 year old girl came into our clinic at the request of her pediatrician. Apparently her mother, Mrs. Fender, had contacted the doctor for a refill of the medication Marianne took for hyperactivity. Mrs. Fender also complained that, because the drugs "no longer worked as well," she found herself needing to constantly increase the amount of medication Marianne received.

The pediatrician, concerned about potential abuse of the medication, suggested that Marianne be re-evaluated before further medications were prescribed. At the time of referral, Marianne was on a dose of medication that was four to five times the amount typically administered to an 11 year old of her height and weight. Mrs. Fender claimed that this level of medication was necessary to maintain "some sanity" at home. According to mother, Marianne was constantly "sassing" her and refusing to do her chores.

At school, Marianne had consistently performed well. She was in the high reading group and had recently been selected for a special science program that was organized for children who demonstrated particular aptitude in that realm. The teachers did note that Marianne seemed to be looking more tired and "dazed" in recent months.

The more we talked with Mrs. Fender, Marianne, and the school, the more it became evident that the girl's problems were confined to the home. Marianne and her mother had an angry relationship which turned particularly sour upon Mr. Fender's departure from home when his daughter was 6 years old. Marianne had always been "Daddy's girl" and, in fact, resembled him physically. Of the three children, she reacted most negatively to her parents' separation and seemed to blame her mother for the breakup. Mrs. Fender alternated between acts of rage and feelings of intense guilt when she dealt with Marianne. When she described the situation to her pediatrician (5 years prior to our evaluation), he suggested that the girl might benefit from medication. Over time, Mrs. Fender began to rely on the medication as a means of attempting to control her daughter's outbreaks of upset and anger. In many ways, Mrs. Fender found it easier to dole out the medication than to set appropriate limits around her daughter's misbehavior.

As part of our evaluation, we tested Marianne both while she was medicated and also when she was off the medication. Our findings indicated that the medication did not appreciably change her performance on any of the tests. Reports from the school on special rating scales were the same regardless of Marianne's drug status. We eventually recommended to Mrs. Fender that she consider family counseling so that she might learn non-chemical approaches to managing her daughter's behavior. We suggested that her daughter's problems might best be understood as something other than ADHD/Hyperactivity. Fortunately, Mrs. Fender responded to our recommendations, although with considerable trepidation.

Each one of the cases described above represents an instance of a child's behavior being "misread" as hyperactivity. These examples should not be understood as reasons for scuttling evaluations of hyperactive behavior or treatment with medication. They are intended to emphasize that: **all that is hyper is not hyperactivity.**

So What Is ADHD/Hyperactivity?

Rather than spit out definitions and criteria for ADHD/Hyperactivity or attempt to describe a "standard" ADHD child (he doesn't exist), we want to review some of the research evidence that underlies our current understanding of the disorder. Don't worry, we won't string you along forever before providing more concrete answers. Our experience, however, is that you will better understand definitions if you first have an idea of their scientific origin.

Problems deciding whom to identify as hyperactive have by no means been limited to parents, schools and physicians. Researchers initially approached the study of hyperactivity by searching for a group of symptoms that characterized the disorder. They developed long lists of supposedly characteristic symptoms ranging from school problems and changing moods to peer problems, aggression, and irritability. Unfortunately, by the time they were finished identifying all the possible behaviors, the only children who weren't described by at least some of the symptoms were three profoundly well-behaved children located somewhere in British Columbia! Most children, at least for periods of time or in particular settings, can act in a rather inattentive, impulsive and hyperactive manner. Forty percent of all four year olds are described by their mothers as hyperactive. Somewhere between 25% and 35% of all 6-8 year old boys are described by their parents as impulsive and overactive. Using the official criteria established by the American Psychiatric Association, we would identify somewhere around 20% of all children 6-8 years of age as hyperactive. Do we really want to label so many of our youth as having a handicapping condition?

We know that children can be "hyper" for all kinds of reasons: children who are caught in the middle of a difficult divorce situation are famous for being distractible and fidgety. Very anxious children are often unable to sit in their seats for long periods of time. Children whose parents do an inadequate job of setting clear limits and establishing consistent consequences for misbehavior tend to exhibit problems with impulse control. Children who are upset, especially young boys, tend to express their worries through physical behavior. Children who are in educational settings which conflict with their own learning style will often attend poorly and underachieve academically. Are all these children hyperactive?

Part of the quandary is that we're trying to get hold of behaviors that can occur as a consequence of normal development, external events, or as a result of other sorts of problems. Also, children by nature are "moving targets" and don't behave with anything approaching consistency from situation to situation, parent to parent, teacher to teacher, day to day. Have you ever come out of a school conference concerning one of your nonhyperactive children seriously wondering if the teacher was describing your child? How many times have you wanted to stop the teacher in the middle of describing this perfect angel and make sure she was talking about the same child who just did his best to redecorate the living room wall with his brother's face?

Unfortunately, ADHD/Hyperactivity has become somewhat of a catch-all label for almost any child who exhibits some kind of disruptive or noncompliant behavior. In our own experience, we have seen a vast range of educational and psychological problems all referred to us with a label of "hyperactivity." This is especially the case after a Phil Donahue has yet another expert on hyperactivity reel off symptoms and cures.

How can we distinguish between the hyperactive child and one who looks hyperactive but isn't? Clues that help to answer that key question have been uncovered when researchers tried to understand why hyperactive children were so seemingly unpredictable. While the behavior of ADHD/Hyperactive children is generally impulsive and out-of-bounds, it is often not consistently abnormal. As one parent described her son, "The only consistency about David is that he is never consistent in the way he behaves." ADHD/Hyperactive children tend to keep their parents and teachers guessing. A teacher once commented to us that her ADHD students seemed to be under some mysterious and unfathomable influence which was beyond her comprehension.

The intense unpredictability of an ADHD child's performance makes it even more understandable that a parent or teacher would quickly adopt the "Lazy Brat" hypothesis to explain a child's poor behavior. After all, here's this normal-looking child with at least average intelligence who one day gets a "100" on a spelling test and the next day behaves as if he were raised in Madagascar and had never seen an English spelling list in his life. "I just know he can do the work," teachers will say, "but something gets in the way. He probably is just too interested in socializing and doesn't really care about academic achievement."

Are ADHD/Hyperactive children totally unpredictable? Not really. While they certainly show inconsistency in their behavior, ADHD/Hyperactive children are not as mysterious as we once believed. A series of research studies conducted over the past ten years has helped us to understand some of the vagaries of hyperactive behavior.

One of the most telling studies was conducted by Dr. Mary Ann Roberts and her colleagues. The purpose of the research project was to compare hyperactive and nonhyperactive boys across three different settings. In the "free play" condition, each child was brought individually to a playroom and told that he could play with whatever he liked for a period of 15 minutes. Behind a one-way mirror, trained observers coded various aspects of the child's behavior, including attention span, on-task behavior, fidgetiness, and the amount of movement. The observers were "blind" to a child's group status (i.e., they did not know which children had been classified as hyperactive and which as nonhyperactive). The children also wore watches which were modified to measure levels of activity.

In the "restricted play" condition, children were again shown the playroom but this time told to sit at one table and play only with a particular toy car. Observers once again recorded characteristics of the child's behavior during that period.

Finally, in the "restricted academic" condition the child was shown around the "classroom" and then directed to a desk. The child was presented with two pencils and five pages of arithmetic problems selected so that they were at a level of difficulty one grade lower than each subject's current grade placement. The examiner completed one problem on each page and then told the child to stay at his desk and work on the remaining problems. As soon as the examiner left, observers began coding the child's behavior.

The results of this project are illuminating. In the "free play" condition, hyperactive children were rated similarly to the nonhyperactive children. In a situation which made few demands for attention and self-control, both groups were relatively comparable across a broad range of behavior ratings. However, as the situation became more restrictive and demanded adherence to rules, the two groups became increasingly distinguishable.

The greatest differences between hyperactive and nonhyperactive children occurred in the restrictive academic condition. The hyperactive children demonstrated a significantly shorter attention span, greater restlessness, and more activity than boys in the nonhyperactive group. Thus, the hyperactive boy's impulsive and inattentive behavior became more pronounced as the environment became more restrictive and rule-oriented. The results of this study mirror comments by parents that their ADHD children would be fine if: 1) They didn't have to go to school, and 2) they didn't have to adhere to other than easily manageable limits (such as "Don't leave the state when you're playing outside").

A study by Drs. James Tallmadge and Russell A. Barkley provides further insights into the nature of hyperactive behavior. In this study mothers and fathers were observed interacting with their hyperactive and nonhyperactive children. One observer coded the parents' behavior in response to a specific behavior of the child, while another observer coded the child's response to a parental behavior. Half the parents and children were ushered into a playroom and told to play freely together. The remaining parents were instructed to work with their children on a set of math problems and drawings.

Interestingly, there were no differences between mothers and fathers in terms of how they interacted with their children. Parents of hyperactive children, however, responded differently to their boys than did parents of nonhyperactive children. The patterns of interaction also depended on whether they occurred in the free play or restricted academic setting. Parents of hyperactive boys gave more commands than parents of nonhyperactive boys, especially in the "task" condition. In response to those commands, the hyperactive boys were more negative and disobedient than the nonhyperactive boys. The hyperactive boys responded differently, though, depending on which parent gave the command (even though parents were similar in their command giving). The hyperactive boys were more negative and less responsive to their mothers' directions than were nonhyperactive boys. In response to their fathers' commands, the hyperactive boys were not different in their responses from the nonhyperactive boys.

Even though parents of hyperactive children became more directive and controlling as the situation changed from the free play to the academic setting, the boys increased their problematic behavior only in response to the mother. This study, among other things, seems to confirm the complaints of many mothers of hyperactive boys that their children tend to behave better in the presence of father. It also demonstrates that the behavior of hyperactive boys is at least somewhat dependent on characteristics of the setting and the nature of adult interaction.

These sorts of findings help to explain how parents and teachers can provide clinicians with starkly contrasting descriptions of a child's status. It is not at all unusual for a parent to arrive at our clinic thoroughly incensed by the school's insistence that they pursue an ADHD evaluation. They will complain bitterly about lousy teachers and schools that are more interested in labeling kids as impaired than in providing good education. They will tell us, "Nothing's wrong with my kid. We have no real problems with him in our home."

When we inquire further and ask what he does upon arrival from the school bus we are told, "He throws his books down on the floor, grabs a cookie and dashes out the door to play." When we ask about meals, "We don't make him sit with us because he fidgets terribly in his chair, gets out of his seat every ten seconds to run for juice or check out a noise in the living room, or change channels on the TV a million times. And he interrupts conversations so much that it's just better if he eats when he's done playing. What we do is leave a dish out for him." (We always wonder if there's a bowl on the floor for the cat, one for the dog, and a plate nearby for the child.)

"How about chores?," we ask. "Not worth it," we'll often hear in reply. "By the time I yell at him a million times to make his bed, it's easier to do it myself. Besides, getting Johnny to finish making his bed can take a lifetime. He'll start to pull the sheet up and then he might see a bird outside his window, so he'll go to the window and maybe see an eraser he likes to play with and before you know it he's in his sister's room looking for some paper to write on and at that point, Doctor, making his bed is just about the farthest thing from his mind — with the possible exception of doing his homework."

We forge ahead, "How about going out shopping or to dinner?" "No way," comes the response. "At the mall he'll dash off in one direction or another, not to defy us but because he sees something of interest and off he goes without stopping a second to remember what we told him about staying near. In fact, when we yell at him for running off, he kind of looks at us with this hurt expression like, 'How was I supposed to stop myself?' As for restaurants, we're pretty much stuck with order-out pizza and the drive-thru at McDonald's. Last time we went out to a real dinner was for Mothers' Day and that experience just about made me want to give up on motherhood altogether. But listen, he's a good kid, a typical busy boy who doesn't want to be trouble, and we've learned how to deal with him. The school is trying to make him out to be some kind of problem but he's really not hyperactive."

If you don't put an ADHD child in a situation that requires attention and compliance to rules, you will not see dramatic differences in his behavior compared to that of other children. Some parents have compensated for their child's impulsiveness and distractibility by adjusting their family's lifestyle to minimize situations bound to cause problems. As we all know, however, school programs cannot provide the same level of flexibility and compensation. They need to sit the child down for assignments and lessons, and will inevitably feel the brunt of the child's attention deficits.

We should also point out that other studies have demonstrated that the tendency of mothers of hyperactive children to be more commanding, negative and controlling seems largely in response to their children's hyperactivity. When hyperactive boys are successfully medicated, their mothers tend to react much more like other mothers. This is an important finding to keep in mind when the parent of a hyperactive child inevitably begins to feel "it's all my fault."

While parents of hyperactive children may well handle situations in ways that exacerbate problem behavior, they are never the "cause" of the problem, *per se*. Ample evidence suggests that parents of hyperactive youngsters behave in ways that are in large part reactive to their children's behavior. This finding lends further credence to the notion that mental illness is hereditary and that we get it from our children!

One more example will help provide clues to the nature of hyperactive behavior. ADHD/Hyperactive children have routinely performed poorly on boring, repetitive tasks that are unrewarding. For example, on tests that require them to be alert to important cues that are embedded in unimportant information, hyperactive children will tend to miss the cues and engage in behavior that is irrelevant to the task at hand.

One such measure which has been used extensively in ADHD/Hyperactivity research is called the "Continuous Performance Test." While there are many versions of this procedure, they all require the child to sit for a period of time in front of a display. Numbers or letters flash on the screen one at a time and the child is told to press the button when a particular sequence appears. No feedback is given to the child upon a correct or incorrect response. While nonhyperactive children find this a relatively easy task, hyperactive children often fail to respond to the target sequence and press the button at the wrong times. If the situation is changed such that separate lights shine upon a correct or incorrect response, the performance of hyperactive children improves significantly. In other words, if the situation provides constant and immediate feedback, the behavior of hyperactive children will become more normal.

Again, the ADHD child's responsiveness to clearly-stated rules as well as to immediate, consistent and meaningful consequences helps to explain why different adults involved with him can often come up with such different descriptions of the same child. In our clinic we recently had a case in which one teacher rated the child as grossly abnormal while another judged the exact same student to be absolutely normal, although perhaps a tad restless. The parents assumed that the teacher offering the positive picture was just a better teacher who knew how to handle kids and was simply more competent. Closer examination suggested an alternative explanation. The teacher who expressed serious concerns about Matt had him for math, language arts and homeroom. Each of the classes had roughly 28 children in them, four or five of whom were "terrors." Math and language arts required a considerable degree of sustained attention and persistence, and, in the case of homeroom, the ability to get oneself organized for the day and stay out of trouble.

In contrast, the other teacher had Matt for a special social studies class that had only 12 children enrolled and was designed largely around class discussion and hands-on projects. Little seatwork was required and a student teacher was involved to help the teacher run the program. Matt loved this class because it engendered few demands for sitting still and the subject was presented in a stimulating and novel fashion. He also told us that the assistant was always nearby to keep him on track. ADHD youngsters will be at their best in one-to-one situations that are highly compelling.

What then are the key characteristics that distinguish between a child with a "true blue" attention deficit and all those children who can look hyperactive but are not? As the studies mentioned above illustrate, the answers seem to lie in the ADHD child's chronic and pervasive inability to organize and control his behavior in routine situations requiring adherence to rules. In the words of Dr. Virginia Douglas, children with a *bona fide* attention deficit, whether they want to or not, simply don't seem to have it in them to "stop, look, listen and think" before responding in situations which require attentiveness and self-control. ADHD children are missing the controls that would help them refrain from leaping before they look. This inability to follow rules and exert self-control starts early in life and manifests itself to some extent in almost all daily activities involving rules and where there are not clear and meaningful external consequences for behavior. Even when he tries hard, the child with this impulsive style seems to be missing the internal brakes necessary to hold off behavior long enough to make good decisions about how to act.

To illustrate these qualities, here's what a teacher wrote about eight year old Ricky:

Ricky's behavior seriously inhibits his academic performance. He is often very distractible and unable to remain on task for long periods of time. Ricky also gets involved in inappropriate activities with other students, such as making noises, talking, and disrupting the class by tapping his pen or stomping his feet.

Ricky often loses credit for lack of organization or for losing work even after it is finished. He does not take responsibility for his work and depends on teachers to keep track of what he has to do. We don't see him as openly defying us. Actually, he's a sweet and loving little boy. It's just that he seems to find it nearly impossible to sit still and follow directions that have multiple steps without him getting lost in another activity. His father calls him a "worm in hot ashes" and that's

28

a fair description of Ricky. I think Ricky has a great deal of academic potential that is hindered by the inconsistencies of his behavior.

Even though Ricky is almost always "busy," there are times when he only needs a few reminders to get back to work. On these days, Ricky is able to complete his assignments with ease, and he even uses free time appropriately. For the life of me, I can't find any rhyme or reason to the pattern of good and bad days.

What underlies the ADHD child's inattention and impulsive style? Is there a primary characteristic that accounts for most of the ADHD symptoms and helps us understand the central nature of the disorder?

ADHD Children Have a Thick Barrier Between Themselves and Life's Many Consequences

To our way of thinking, the best way to understand the essence of ADHD is to keep in mind the notion of a "thick barrier" that stands firmly between the child and the various efforts on the part of the outside world to exert appropriate influence and control over his behavior. The rewards, punishments, and incentives which usually make it through a child's skull and influence behavior seem to bounce off the ADHD child's thick barrier. It's as if their microphone is turned down so far that instructions and consequences aren't received "loud and clear." Even when the message gets through, its impact is not felt for long. When we discuss non-medical treatment approaches, we will be talking about the need to develop programs which are designed to make it through the barrier.

The concept of a biologically-based thick barrier helps to understand many of the primary problems associated with ADHD. A leading researcher and proponent of a thick barrier hypothesis, Dr. Russell Barkley of the University of Massachusetts Medical Center, summarized the core problems this way:

Primary Deficits of ADHD/Hyperactive Children

1. Unable to cope with routine rules

2. Unable to sustain appropriate behavior in the absence of clear, frequent and immediate consequences

3. Effects of rewards and punishments wear off quickly

These deficits all concern the ADHD child's inherent difficulties in being appropriately regulated by his environment. An ADHD child falters when confronted with rules, moves away from tasks unless there are very clear limits for and immediate consequences to behavior, and needs reinforcements that are always interesting or meaningful. In situations where there are few rules or where limits are clear as well as intensely reinforced, the ADHD child will evidence far less problematic behavior.

Incidentally, you will again notice that the characteristics outlined by Dr. Barkley are more related to the quality of a hyperactive child's behavior than to the sheer quantity of activity. In many ways the term "hyperactivity" is unfortunate because we have made far more progress in understanding the disorder by studying the "how" of the hyperactive child's behavior than the "how much." Keys to unlocking some of the intricacies of ADHD/Hyperactivity have usually been discovered when we have tried to explore the nature of a hyperactive child's interactions with the world, rather than when we have simply measured levels of activity.

While we have discussed at some length the first two characteristics described by Dr. Barkley, the third deficit may require more clarification. To the great frustration of parents with a hyperactive child, rewards and punishments seem to have an unusually limited effect on the child's behavior. Whereas a scolding might keep a nonhyperactive child well-behaved for most of a day, it might only "work" on the hyperactive child for a few minutes before more misbehavior ensues. For some children, rewards with stars or small gifts can have a longstanding impact on their behavior. ADHD/ Hyperactive children seem to lose interest in the reward program after only a few days. In psychological terms, they "habituate" to positive or negative reinforcement far more rapidly than their nonhyperactive peers. Just when the parent of a hyperactive child thinks he or she has a system that is motivating, the rewards or punishments seem to lose their appeal. Unfortunately, rather than change to another set of reinforcements, parents understandably become frustrated and surrender.

Another important concept that helps to differentiate between the true ADHD child and children who look hyperactive but most likely are not rests in what Dr. Jan Loney of Stony Brook University calls the "can't versus won't" dimension. While the ADHD child can be willful, he often has trouble with self-control, sustained attention, and organization even when he wants to do well. You have the sense with the ADHD child that he often cannot attend or delay for love nor money except in unique situations which are rich in feedback and consequences.

Parents of one hyperactive child told us that their son, Tommy, often seemed as mystified as they when he got into trouble. One day they allowed him to ride his bike on the driveway with the clear understanding that he needed to stop his bike at the edge of the pavement so that he would not disturb a newly-seeded patch of grass. Tommy said that he would do his best to stay off the grass since he had himself helped to plant the seeds and had been watching them carefully as they began to grow. Within ten minutes of riding, however, only a few blades of grass still remained unscathed. When his father asked him why he did not stop himself in time, Tommy said, "I would ride around and before I knew it, there I was on the grass." Tommy's father said that he believed the sincerity of his son's account. As he put it, "Tommy just gets out of control of Tommy." This boy, like many ADHD/Hyperactive children, often misbehaved not out of willful opposition to authority but because his impulses got the best of him.

Conversely, the hyper-but-not-hyperactive child often shows the capacity for self-control but chooses, either consciously or otherwise, to resist demands for adherence to rules. With the troublesome–but–non-hyperactive–child there is evidence that he "has it in him" to attend and plan, but that something gets in the way of successful performance. Perhaps the child is distracted by concerns about peer acceptance or by a father's alcoholism or mother's unhappiness or a brother's predominance. Maybe the child is too angry to concentrate on school work or is highly oppositional or rarely has had the experience of suffering a consequence for misbehavior or is so fearful of failing that he chooses to avoid demands by running from them. It is also possible that the child suffers from a specific learning disability that causes him to struggle in school and to experience failure and frustration. Again, a child can appear hyperactive for many reasons, but only a relative few experience the kinds of pervasive difficulties that are associated with ADHD/Hyperactivity.

Incorporating some of these concepts, researchers have been attempting to establish criteria that will limit the identification of ADHD/Hyperactivity to just those children with a longstanding impulsive and/or inattentive style. Much research has been devoted to developing ways to assess some of the characteristics we have discussed. As you will appreciate, the evaluation of children referred for hyperactivity needs to be a comprehensive effort. Information must be gathered across a variety of situations and from different people involved in the child's life. As you also know, most hyperactive children are not themselves very open and reflective about their problems or necessarily motivated to seek help. We have yet to receive a call from a hyperactive child who says, "I would like to make an appointment to discuss my hyperactive behavior!!"

Researchers have now produced increasingly accurate tools and techniques for the assessment of ADHD/Hyperactivity. They have developed rating scales that help to ensure that the child's problems do indeed concern issues of attention and impulsivity. They have also developed tests to document that the impulsivity and inattentiveness occur to an abnormal degree, and we make sure that the hyperactive behavior didn't just appear overnight or last month.

Simply stated, we have developed protocols which address the following questions: 1) What's the problem? 2) When did it start? 3) How bad is it? 4) How consistently has it presented itself? and 5) How pervasively does it affect the child's life? The practitioner and researcher also try to rule out other possible explanations for the child's behavior such as mental retardation (IQ below 70), severe speech and language delays, brain damage, severe emotional problems, etc. Not everyone agrees on what the best measures are or where cutoffs for abnormality should be set, but we seem to be making progress in arriving at some agreement about meaningful criteria. As you will learn in the next chapter, however, ADHD/Hyperactivity is not a unitary entity. Even children who clearly meet these criteria differ from one another in some important ways.

PRINCIPLE 4

There Is No Such Thing as THE Hyperactive Child

Even when we use scientific criteria to select "truly ADHD" children, we still identify a mixed bag of children. For some reason your children do not read the official criteria before they behave the way they do. As such, one ADHD child can behave very differently from other ADHD children and still be ADHD. You can't talk about **the** hyperactive child any more than you can talk about **the** diabetic child. We know that there are different forms of diabetes and that each requires different treatment approaches.

We are coming to grips with the fact that, similarly, there are various subgroups of ADHD/Hyperactive children and that each requires tailored approaches to treatment. Children differ in the degree to which they exhibit those impulsive, inattentive behaviors. They also spice the brew with different amounts of other qualities. When we evaluate a child for ADHD/Hyperactivity, we first check to make sure he has that chronic impulsive style and then we see how he falls along other important dimensions of behavior.

Once the clinician feels convinced that the child has ADHD/Hyperactivity, it becomes necessary to determine whether or not the child, in addition to his attention deficit, is physically impulsive and overactive. Children who are both inattentive **and** physically impulsive, as a group, experience more academic and social problems, and are often more difficult to treat. Because he represents more of a problem to parents and teachers, however, the overactive, impulsive child sometimes gets help more quickly than the inattentive but relaxed child (often a girl) who can be dubbed a "daydreamer" or "social butterfly" and get overlooked. The silently inattentive child is more likely to be considered underachieving because of family and motivational problems. Indeed, many children who are normally-active and inattentive do in fact suffer from problems not associated with ADHD. But some of these youngsters find sustaining attention to be a near impossible act regardless of their emotional status or family situation.

Don't forget that a child (and adult for that matter) can be highly impulsive and disinhibited in non-physical ways. Some children may not physically be all over the house or classroom but show little capacity to control what comes out of their mouths. One mother of an 11-year old boy recently marveled at his ability to blurt out absolutely anything and everything that came into his mind regardless of the social consequences. His barrage of questions and comments was forever driving family members to distraction and creating embarrassing situations. Chris could always be counted on to say just the wrong thing in the presence of a less-than-favored relative or obese individual at the grocery store, not because he was especially mean-spirited, but because he would give little thought to the impact of his words. As his mother put it, "The thought strikes, the words come out, and nothin' stands in their way."

Sometimes impulsiveness manifests itself primarily in the way in which an individual processes information. The father of an ADHD child could empathize with his son's frustrations around neatly and accurately completing written work because father, too, had a life-long tendency to let his mind "race ahead of my hand." "It happens all the time at work," he told us. "I'll start writing and the sentences will pour into my head and, because I can't slow down, I'll be three sentences ahead of where I'm writing. I'm in such a rush to get the words down that I don't go back to check what I've written, which usually is a terrible mess. I've tried all sorts of strategies to write at a more even pace, but I always find myself losing control and getting increasingly frustrated. I may start out okay, but by the end of the first paragraph, it's not a pretty sight. Thank heavens for competent secretaries!"

Because the compliant but inattentive child usually is not the classroom's squeakiest wheel, he or she is often identified as ADHD at a later age and, unfortunately, after much opportunity for intervention has passed. (Psychological testing of the sort we will describe under Principle 9 is especially useful in identifying the inattentive-but-not-overactive child.) So keep in mind:

You Don't Need To Be Darting Across the Ceilings To Be Considered an ADHD/Hyperactive Child

After considering issues related to activity level and physical impulsiveness, the practitioner next seeks to assess whether or not the child is also aggressive and/or oppositional. Some hyperactive children, because of frustration, low self-esteem, or other issues, are quite angry and will harm themselves or others. Thus, in addition to their primary attention deficit, they exhibit high levels of angry and, at times, delinquent behavior. Others may not be physically aggressive but are unusually oppositional. Even when asked to do something well within their capabilities, they, seemingly on principle, automatically and stubbornly refuse. Children who are both ADHD/Hyperactive and aggressive or oppositional are the most difficult to treat because they often behave in ways that frustrate or anger parents, teachers and

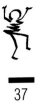

mental health professionals. Frankly, aggressive children are also more likely to have parents who have short fuses and/or who are prone to act out their anger and frustrations physically. Such parents are often hard to work with because they can become easily threatened and angered.

We have found it important, though, to make sure that behavior reported as aggressive is truly a byproduct of anger and hostile intent as opposed to yet another consequence of the child's impulsiveness. An actual clinical example best illustrates the point: One of our ADHD patients was suspended from school for hitting the gym teacher and another child in the class. We were surprised because Josh impressed us as an unusually carefree and loving child who, if anything, too often allowed himself to be the brunt of other children's barbs.

When we talked with Josh and then his teacher, it became clear that poor self-control and not aggression was the culprit in this situation. Josh and the rest of his class were running laps around the gym. At one point he saw one of his friends stick his arms out like an airplane and make propeller noises. Thinking this looked like fun, Josh immediately shot his own arms out in preparation for takeoff. Unfortunately, he didn't stop to consider that his teacher and a little boy were in his flight path and not particularly pleased to be clobbered by the left wing. He was then grounded for three days because of his "aggressive behavior." Josh was mystified and saddened by this incident because his intentions were not at all aggressive.

The ADHD child's impulsiveness always seems to put him in compromising situations. A father once told us, "Ten boys might be flinging mashed potatoes with their spoons, but sure as the sun shines it will be my son who gets caught and punished. You see, all the other kids have the sense to check first to make sure that none of the teachers are watching. Not Jason. He'll launch the potatoes first and then turn around to find the principal glaring at him. At this point, it's just assumed in that school that if there's trouble, there's Jason. The kid doesn't stand a chance." ADHD children are indeed the most inept of criminals. What gets in the way of good school performance also hinders successful mischief.

Of concern to parents and educators is that ADHD children will often make up lame excuses and transparent lies when confronted with misdeeds. They worry that, not only do they have a disruptive child on their hands, they also have to deal with a sociopath who lies at the drop of a hat. If you examine the situation surrounding the lie, however, it often becomes more understandable and a little less alarming: ADHD Johnny is walking down the hallway and sees an open gym locker. Without thinking and with good intention, he slams the door shut, only to hear the ear-piercing scream from the youngster who was behind the door putting books away.

Mayhem ensues. A frustrated teacher grabs Johnny by the arm and drags him to the principal's office. This is the third time in as many days that the principal has to deal with this youngster's reckless behavior and he's not happy. "Why did you hurt that little girl in the hallway?," he thunders. Johnny is cornered once again. He's not sure why he slammed the door. It was just there and he didn't think much about it. He knows that he's in big trouble and that, given his numerous offenses over the past few days, his chances of Dad taking him to the baseball game are becoming slim. He's never been good at reasoned conversation (especially under pressure) so he blurts out, "But it wasn't me! You see, it looked like me but it was really James who was walking behind me..." and out pours this poorly thought out story that convinces no one. Before you know it, he's in trouble not only for slamming the door but also for telling the most improbable story ever concocted.

ADHD children are forever getting into trouble, sometimes with malice aforethought but often because of their inattention and poor impulse control. Understandably, they can become frustrated with always being fingered for one misdeed or another. So what happens? They fall into the habit of impulsively lying about their responsibility in the hope that they can deflect some of the heat that all too frequently comes their way. It's always someone else's fault. Our intention is not to excuse all the misbehavior of ADHD children as merely a byproduct of their handicap. And we certainly are not implying that it be dismissed without consequence. We are simply suggesting that parents and teachers keep in mind that lying and cheap excuses can be more an ADHD child's desperate and impulsive attempt to avoid punishment than the devilish plans of a master criminal trying to pull one over on the authorities.

Our next goal in the diagnostic process is to evaluate the degree to which the child's attention deficit is exacerbated by behavior problems that are not wholly tied to impulsiveness. Some ADHD children display conduct problems that go well beyond the sort of impulsive behaviors associated with ADHD/Hyperactivity. They may engage in particularly disruptive or manipulative behavior that they plan out to some degree. They may work out a scheme with their buddies to steal something or skip school or deface property. This sort of behavior can emanate from an environment that is unusually inconsistent or even chaotic. Not only does that child get into trouble out of his impulsiveness, he also has few models in his environment that can show him how to deal with limits and frustrations. Children don't arrive in the world fully aware of all the rules and regulations. They need to be taught appropriate behavior and have the opportunity to experience consistent consequences surrounding their actions. Because some ADHD youngsters live in unpredictable and/or lax environments, they also develop conduct problems in their own right. As we've said repeatedly, ADHD is not caused by bad parenting or teaching, but it sure can be made worse by them. In our attempts to arrive at reasonable recommendations, then, it helps us to know whether, in addition to the attention deficits, there are specific behavior problems that require treatment in their own right.

Incidentally, we've been impressed by the fact that inconsistency and chaos can occur in the "best" of homes. We have been thinking that there should be a "Yuppie Deficit Disorder" to describe children with parents who are so busy with high-pressure careers (and guilt-ridden when they come home) that they rarely take the opportunity to set and enforce rules.

A five year old boy was referred for kicking and biting his parents, both of whom were prominent and highly intelligent professionals. The problems would usually occur when he was told to get ready for bed or pick up his toys. When asked how they handled these situations, they told us that they would sit him down and, in their most sensitive and growth-promoting tones (not wanting to inhibit his emotional expressiveness, creativity or self-esteem), would discuss at length the many consequences of his actions. The little boy would hear about how his kicking made Mommy and Daddy feel, and what could happen to his chances of worldly success if he continued to kick, and why society cannot tolerate outbursts in its citizens. Did the child ever experience a meaningful and tangible consequence for his misbehavior? Never.

In a misguided effort to avoid conflict and punishment, some parents never help their offspring learn that some things they do are wrong and will invariably be met with dire consequences.

PRINCIPLE 5

Find a Clinician Who Works Closely With the School

ADHD/Hyperactivity has a powerful impact on a child's educational adjustment. The symptoms invariably surface in the school setting and significantly impair achievement. In fact, many see ADHD/Hyperactivity as essentially a psychoeducational disturbance. Teachers are therefore a crucial source of information about many of the areas associated with attention deficits. A teacher can report on how the child attends in class, gets along with peers, responds to structure, handles transition periods, and acquires academic skills. Yet for reasons that are hard for us to fathom, many clinicians have little if any contact with the school, despite the wealth of information available from that source. Unfortunately, it is far more novel than typical for a school to hear from a clinician involved with a family seeking services for ADHD. Poor communication between your practitioner and the school will inevitably make it harder to evaluate and treat your child.

While clinicians usually have a general theoretical orientation to the management of mental health problems, most are willing to fit the treatment to the problem (rather than the other way around). For example, a clinician might tend to view and treat most problems in the context of family functioning, but nonetheless engage a patient in individual psychotherapy when the situation demands. You will find some clinicians who have a relatively fixed approach to managing nearly all mental health problems. Some deal with all childhood disorders essentially as manifestations of family disturbance and spend relatively limited time evaluating the child in his own right. From their perspective, the therapist's primary role is to help the family better handle conflicts that arise, by altering the family's system of assuming roles and relating to one another. Family therapists, as a group, are more invested in encouraging the family to advocate for themselves than they are oriented toward ongoing professional consultation to schools.

Some clinicians, on the other hand, deal with child mental health problems as largely a byproduct of inner psychological conflict around such issues as early relationships to parents and comfort with sexual or aggressive impulses. Their focus on resolving internal conflict through techniques aimed at helping the child gain personal awareness tends to reduce investment in dealing directly with more external events, such as school functioning. Finally, some of the professionals who become involved in the diagnosis of ADHD take a strictly medical or neurological approach to the disorder and, as a consequence, view the child's behavior in different settings as primarily an outgrowth of biological events which the clinician seeks to analyze and alter. This orientation, when adopted wholeheartedly, also tends to diminish the importance of school-based intervention.

We want to make it clear that all the approaches mentioned above are thoroughly legitimate models for managing mental health problems and, indeed, can play important roles in the diagnosis and treatment of ADHD/Hyperactivity. Our concern revolves around the extent to which some practitioners limit their involvement with schools (and sometimes parents) because they adhere to approaches that focus on only one level of a problem. From our perspective, ADHD is a highly complex disorder which works its way into all levels of a child's experience and represents more than simply family dysfunction, inner conflict, or neurological pathology. As such, we feel that the most effective clinicians are those who are willing to gather information from multiple sources and arrive at diagnostic decisions based not upon theoretical bias but upon a reasonable integration of data. For this sort of chronic and multi-faceted disorder, you will need someone who is willing and able to get involved with the diversity of issues that inevitably arises at home, in school and within the community.

You will notice we are not advocating that you seek out professionals from any particular discipline. We do not feel that only a pediatrician or psychologist or psychiatrist or neurologist can handle referrals for ADHD appropriately. In our experience, competence in this area is far more a matter of attitude and specific training in the area of ADHD than of professional background, *per se.* We have seen credible evaluations conducted by practitioners from all the major disciplines and, conversely, we have been appalled at some of the ill-informed and flippant opinions rendered by highly-regarded professionals.

Part of the message we wish to convey is that you need to take an active and forceful role in securing the best available professional help and in working confidently with that professional. You need to pose hard questions, be willing to challenge or at least ask about those things you are unsure of, and, in essence, become an active collaborator in the process. When you first meet a clinician, ask whether or not he has had specific training in the diagnosis and treatment of ADHD/ Hyperactivity. Does he regularly attend professional workshops on this topic? How many patients has he evaluated for this disorder? How involved does he become in monitoring treatment programs? How available is he if there's a problem?

You should feel comfortable working with practitioners and should not remain in situations where pro-
nouncements come from on high, or your concerns are
dismissed out of hand. Clinicians tend to get most de-
fensive and arrogant when they are least sure of themselves. If you are uncomfortable with a practitioner's approach or personal style, either confront him or her
directly about your concerns or find someone else. Pas-
sivity will get you nowhere in this process. Close contact with the school is one of those issues upon which
you should insist.

How Do I Find a Competent Clinician?

Sometimes it's easy because there's a well-regarded
and visible specialty clinic and/or individual practitioner
in your area who has a reputation for state-of-the-art
management of the disorder. Your school or pediatrician
will usually know who offers these kinds of services, and
can make one or more referrals. A parent support group
also tends to keep track of qualified and responsive clinicians. If your community happens to have a medical
center or university, then you might call the department
that houses Child Psychiatry, Child Psychology, or Pedi-
atrics and ask them where such services can be ob-
tained. Lastly, many areas have a mental health bureau
that lists practitioners by specialty area and provides
names of local resources.

If you live in an area where there simply isn't anyone
with specific expertise in handling referrals for ADHD/
Hyperactivity, you may need to take a trip to the closest
available specialist. Most major metropolitan areas have
someone who can provide appropriate services. Clinicians are usually willing, with sufficient notice, to conduct the evaluation in a way that accommodates your

travel schedule. But before packing your suitcase, make sure that help isn't available right in your area. Sometimes parents feel that they can only get sophisticated help by going to an expert out of town, even when competent services are available locally. Being from another city doesn't necessarily bestow upon a clinician greater erudition or skill. There are also real advantages to working with a clinician who is nearby and easily accessible on an ongoing basis.

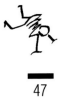

PRINCIPLE 6

Don't Let the Pediatrician Look at Your Child's Angelic Behavior and Call You an Hysteric (Unless It's True)

To the utter bewilderment of mothers, highly active, destructive, and inattentive children have a habit of behaving with exquisite calm and compliance in the pediatrician's office. Yes, the child you just had to pick up from school because he was suspended for pulling the fire alarm and who, five minutes after you brought him home, managed to disassemble your microwave oven ("because he needed the door for a hatch on his play submarine"), smiles angelically at the doctor and makes urbane and pleasant conversation.

The doctor looks at the child and sees a pretty normal-looking kid. He looks at you and sees your eyes bugging out and veins popping from your neck as you become overwhelmed with frustration. The clinician will probably also hear that the child minds better with father than with you, the mother. So he comes to the conclusion that: 1) You don't know how to handle your child, and 2) Johnny doesn't need Ritalin but you might need Valium.

In the trade, this process is known as "parent bashing." The clinician figures that there's nothing wrong with the child so there must be something wrong with the parent. The practitioner's error comes from jumping to conclusions based on observations of nonrepresentative behavior. That's one reason why only 20% of the hyper-active population is diagnosed as such by pediatricians (although physicians are by no means the only poten-tially guilty party).

The flaw surrounding conclusions based on a child's behavior in a doctor's office is that it is an environment which almost ensures the best of behavior from most children. After all, the child is in a one-to-one situation with an adult authority figure. Most children are appre-hensive that, if they act up, they'll get a shot or have to urinate in a cup. Finally, there usually are few demands for sustained attention or self-control during a brief pedi-atric examination. Children who are identified in this kind of setting typically are the most severe and aggres-sive referrals who might have tipped over the fish tank in the waiting room or trashed the doctor's office in the course of the first five minutes.

The point, then, is that a child's behavior in the doc-tor's office is an unreliable indicator of the level and ex-tent of attention deficits. It is also one reason why we suggest that the "Maybe" ADHD/Hyperactive child be tested on objective tests of attention and self-control. Clinicians who say "I know one when I see one" are probably those who are only diagnosing the most severe cases, usually those with a strong aggressive compo-nent. They will tend to miss children, especially girls, whose problems reside more on the side of attention difficulties than of impulsive behavior.

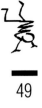

PRINCIPLE 7

Response to Medication Is Not a Valid Measure of ADHD/Hyperactivity

As you will read, stimulant medications can be very useful as **part of the treatment** for ADHD/Hyperactivity. Unfortunately, some clinicians try to judge whether or not a youngster is hyperactive by the child's response to a trial of medication. If the child seems to improve on medications, then the doctor will declare him or her to be ADHD/Hyperactive. In other words, the clinician lets the response to a treatment dictate who is ADHD/Hyperactive and who is not.

Incidentally, this is one way of making a particular treatment 100% effective. What if you only had an ear infection if you responded well to the first antibiotic prescribed? The antibiotic treatment would always be successful because only ear infections that improved with antibiotics would be considered ear infections. The 15% or so of individuals who had ear infections but were not helped by the first antibiotic would be diagnosed as having healthy ears or some other problem. These patients presumably would have some trouble with this practice as deafness approached.

The real flaw in this "Drug as Test" strategy is that we have evidence that all children, and for that matter adolescents and adults, respond to moderate doses of stimulant medication by becoming more attentive and calm. In other words, children other than hyperactive children respond to stimulants in a similar fashion. The response to medication is nondiagnostic. Another problem with the approach is that children respond to the various medications and different dosages in highly individualized ways (you'll read more about this issue shortly). Some very impulsive and inattentive children do not respond to medication at usual doses or perhaps at all. There are good reasons for trials of medication, but medication for the purpose of evaluation is not one of them.

PRINCIPLE 8

An IQ Test Is Not a Valid Measure of ADHD/Hyperactivity

Psychologists, especially school psychologists, put a lot of stock in the standard intelligence test, the Wechsler Intelligence Scale for Children-Revised (WISC-R), for decisions regarding possible ADHD/Hyperactivity. Three subscales on this test (Coding, Digit Span, and Arithmetic) are looked to for information about impulsiveness and distractibility — they form what has been called the "Freedom from Distractibility" factor. There is indeed evidence that ADHD children do poorly on these three subtests. The problem is that so can children with significant learning disabilities, sequencing problems, anxiety disorders, and giftedness. In essence, this factor does not discriminate ADHD/Hyperactive children from other children who have problems of one sort or another.

This is the trouble with using many of the tests in the standard psychological test battery to diagnose ADHD/Hyperactivity. It is in fact true that the hyperactive child's impulsivity will lead to lower scores on most tests. But these tests were not designed to measure attentiveness and self-control **alone** but also other areas, such as visual-motor functioning, intelligence or personality organization. So, for example, poor performance on a Bender Gestalt test, which measures visual-motor functioning (the ability to integrate what you see with what you do with your hands), may be due to impulsivity, but it also can be the result of a significant delay in visual-motor development. In other words, these various tests are not terribly clean or precise measures of attentiveness and self-control. It is hard for the clinician to tease out whether a particular score is the consequence of anxiety, impulsivity, learning problems or normality.

You also are aware by this point that we feel you should be wary of anyone trying to convince you that scores on any one test are sufficient to rule in or out a diagnosis of ADHD/Hyperactivity. Low scores on the Freedom from Distractibility Factor do not an ADHD child make! Test data are a critical component of competent assessment but they cannot be interpreted in isolation.

Despite our cautions about the use of the school psychologists' standard test battery for diagnosis of attention deficits, we want to make it abundantly clear that information generated by psychological testing is of utmost importance in addressing issues relevant to diagnosis and treatment. The test battery represents the best source of data regarding intellectual functioning, visual-motor ability, learning disabilities, and personality style. Furthermore, the school psychologist can often be your best ally in securing and integrating educational services and helping you find your way through bureaucracies. Never underestimate the power of a competent and effective school psychologist. He knows the system and can be of tremendous assistance in arranging, implementing, and monitoring a school program.

Make Sure Your Child's Evaluation Includes an Objective Measure of ADHD/Hyperactivity

Much of our own research has involved developing objective tests of attention and self-control. We were motivated to pursue this project largely out of profound frustration. It bothered us that so much of the evaluation for ADHD/Hyperactivity came either from tests not designed to assess the disorder, or from the subjective reports of parents and teachers. While there is no question that the opinions of parents and teachers are of inestimable value in the evaluative process, it concerned us that such important decisions about a child were based almost entirely upon individual perceptions.

We all have different tolerances for what is too little or too much of a particular behavior. Some of us are more patient than others such that one person's wild child is another's spunky little boy. We often think of the letters that are shown at the end of the TV program *Sixty Minutes*. Some will write that the interviewer was unfair, overly-critical, or downright nasty to a much-maligned individual. Inevitably, the rest will complain that Morley Safer was too lenient or in some fashion coddled a dastardly villain. Yet everybody saw the same show!

It perplexes clinicians when one teacher describes a child as manifesting all the classic symptoms of ADHD/Hyperactivity and then another teacher insists that Johnny is, at worst, a little rambunctious. As we mentioned earlier, parents and teachers often disagree on whether or not a child is hyperactive. In fact, the clinician will hear the same depictions of behavior from home and school in only about one third to one half of all cases. Reasons for the lack of agreement are not hard to fathom: parents and teachers see the child in settings which differ in the degree to which there are expectations for adherence to rules and for sustained attention. For example, some children do better in a school where there is a lot of stimulation and structure than in a home where activities are loosely structured or unexciting. While the differing opinions are very understandable, they place the clinician in the position of not knowing which description of behavior is most representative.

Our concern over the dominance of subjectivity in evaluations led to the development of the Gordon Diagnostic System (GDS). We wanted to include in our evaluations data based on a child's actual behavior in situations requiring delay and sustained attention, but not advanced intellectual abilities or visual-motor skills. The GDS is a portable, electronic device which administers a series of game-like tasks to children. For the Delay Task, the child is told that he will play a game in which he can earn points by pressing a button, waiting a while, and then pressing it again. If he waits long enough before pressing the button, a red light shines and a counter adds one point to his score. If he doesn't wait long enough, the light doesn't shine, no points are recorded, and he has to wait all over again. The computer inside the GDS keeps track of how many times the child pressed the button and the number of correct responses.

Nonhyperactive children find this a very easy task to manage; for the entire eight-minute session they typically press the button, count to between 10 or 20, and then press the button again, count to 10 or 20, press the button, and so forth.. Even four and five year olds wait long enough 80% or 90% of the time. Children with problems of self-control, however, find it hard to cope with this task. They tend to press the button impulsively and have trouble coming up with a strategy for helping themselves wait. Hyperactive children are typically rewarded for only 40% or 50% of their responses. Unlike nonhyperactive children who use an internal means of delaying (i.e., counting to themselves), hyperactive children will tend to engage in some form of physical activity between responses. We have seen children, for example, repeatedly press the button, run around the table five times, then press it again, or talk to the examiner in between each press of the button.

Another "game" administered by the GDS is called the Vigilance Task. The child sees a series of numbers flash one at a time on the screen and is told to press the button every time a "9" comes after a "1." For nine minutes the child has to somehow remain alert to this "hot combination" of digits that appear at irregular intervals. As you might imagine, ADHD children have a terrible time with this task: they will either miss the "1/9" combination or press the button inappropriately. Typically the hyperactive child will press the button on the number following a "1," whether or not it is indeed a "9." In other words, the impulsive child, as intelligent as he or she may be, tends not to wait the extra few milliseconds to make sure that the number that comes right after the "1" is a "9." In many ways, failure on the GDS to inhibit behavior just long enough to behave appropriately is a model for what happens during much of the ADHD child's day and accounts for why this technique has been found to be valid.

In order to standardize the GDS and thereby establish what are normal and abnormal scores, we have tested over 1500 nonhyperactive children aged 4 to 18.

We also have tested over 1000 children who are either hyperactive or experience some other kind of psychiatric disorder, such as severe emotional problems or learning disabilities. The GDS is being used in research and clinical practice in the United States, Canada, and Europe so a great deal of data are being collected on the performance of different groups of children. Importantly, the GDS is being used in the monitoring of stimulant medication therapy. As you will read later, systematic evaluation of drug effects is critical to successful treatment.

The GDS is not presented as some kind of magical device that somehow divines the hyperactive child. We strongly encourage clinicians to conduct a comprehensive evaluation that includes rating scales, interviews, and other testing. We do feel that the GDS provides some information not otherwise available and can help the clinician make a more accurate diagnosis and avoid some of the pitfalls we've discussed. At the least, use of the GDS allows the clinician to see your child under conditions requiring attentiveness and self-control.

It also should be said that a small number of other objective measures are available. Our experience is that these other approaches tend not to be as widely used or well-normed as the GDS. The important thing, though, is that some objective measure be employed in the evaluation.

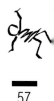

PRINCIPLE 10

Yes, Virginia,
Girls Can Be Hyperactive

In just about any discussion of hyperactivity you will read that this is mainly a disorder of boys. The typical ratios given are anywhere from 6 to 12 hyperactive boys for every hyperactive girl. In other words, the claim is that only about 10% of the hyperactive population is female.

Some of our own research impacts on this issue. In norming and validating the GDS we expected to find some significant differences in scores between boys and girls. After all, a higher percentage of the male population is referred for hyperactivity and everybody knows that girls are more attentive and have better self-control. Imagine our surprise when we found that scores for groups of boys and girls were absolutely identical. As a matter of fact, we have yet to find a sex difference in scores regardless of what group of children we are studying. How can that be?

Other data indicate that ADHD girls, along most dimensions, are similar to ADHD boys in that they perform poorly in school, experience peer problems, and are inattentive. We know that girls identified as hyperactive tend to display their hyperactivity more through attention deficits than through problems with impulsivity and aggression. Hyperactive girls tend not to be as physically active as hyperactive boys and they tend not to show as many conduct problems. This may be why hyperactive girls are often referred for "daydreaming" rather than ADHD/Hyperactivity. They tend not to be as physically unmanageable but certainly can have serious problems sustaining attention and organizing themselves.

Our own belief is that, while we professionals are seriously overdiagnosing hyperactivity in boys, we are just as seriously underdiagnosing the problem in girls. On many occasions our testers have come back in frustration after having tested a little girl whose GDS scores were clearly abnormal, but who was rated by the teacher as nonhyperactive. When asked, the teacher has typically acknowledged that, yes indeed, the girl had trouble attending and completing work. But then the teacher would go on to say that the girl was just a bit of a tomboy and not as hard to handle as some of the boys. As always, squeaky wheels do indeed tend to get the grease.

The area of hyperactivity in girls is just now beginning to get attention from the research community. Over the next few years you may be hearing more about the profile of a hyperactive girl as distinct from the hyperactive boy. The point to you as parents is that sometimes the so-called daydreaming girl is more truly an ADHD child.

PRINCIPLE 11

There's No Better Treatment Than Accurate Diagnosis

We will leave the area of evaluation with just one more reminder about the importance of a sophisticated assessment. While this plea might be viewed as a promotional announcement for those of us involved in psychological evaluations, it is sincerely intended as a reminder of the need for a careful understanding of your child's problems before attempting treatment. You just don't want to find yourself having wasted valuable time and money because of hasty decisions.

Because there are no standard protocols for evaluating ADHD/Hyperactivity, clinicians employ different techniques. Some will rely more heavily on particular rating scales while others stress the importance of interviewing you, the parent. You have read our opinions about essential elements of a comprehensive evaluation. In the least, the assessment should obtain information from the three major sources: you, the school, and your child. Cursory examination of any of these areas heightens the chance of error.

The more systematically information is gathered, the more reliable the evaluation will be. It is for this reason that careful evaluations will use multiple questionnaires as well as the objective tests alongside more informal discussion. The questionnaires usually present a long list of items regarding behavior and physical problems, such as overactivity, fighting, headaches and bedwetting. Your job is to mark those items that describe your child; similar forms are completed by the teacher. It isn't necessary to worry too much about your response to each item. While you obviously should depict your child as accurately as possible, significant errors will not follow from checking that a particular problem occurs "always" instead of "almost always."

The clinician scores these questionnaires and generates a profile of behavior problems for your child. He can get a sense of the range of difficulties exhibited and, because there are norms for how parents of nonhyperactive children rate their youngsters, he can also begin to assess the severity of the problems. It is useful for the clinician to know whether or not your concerns about your child are at a level similar to those of most other parents. Another real advantage to obtaining these ratings is that they can be used to monitor your child's progress in treatment. We, the practitioners, can look at the original, "baseline" scores and determine if treatment, at least from the teacher's or your point of view, has produced any change at all. You'll remember that objective tests can be involved in that same process.

While it may seem that the careful evaluation with its bundle of questionnaires, tests, phone calls, and interviews would take forever to complete, it actually can be managed in a relatively brief period of time. In our clinic, families complete the various written materials and send them to us prior to the first appointment. In that way we can have everything scored and analyzed. We often also have received information from the school and, in most cases, have written material from at least one teacher. When we actually sit down with parents, we already have benefited from a wealth of information.

Individual practitioners have their own style of working with families around interviews and testing. We'll describe our protocol but keep in mind that it is somewhat unique because we are in a medical center setting that stresses research and training.

In our clinic, we first meet with both parents and the child to settle any nerves, discuss how we conduct evaluations, and to answer questions. Then mother and child spend time in our playroom where we can observe them interacting. At the outset they are told that there will be 15 minutes of free play, a five-minute cleanup period, and 15 minutes during which a series of age-appropriate math and letter search worksheets need to be competed.

This observation is not a test of maternal competence! We simply want to see the child "in action" both when rules are at a minimum as well as when there are demands for attending to school materials. It helps us to get a sense of how the child responds to requests for compliance and the sorts of strategies the mother uses if the child refuses to comply. We understand that our observation room is not like your living room and that your child may behave differently in the two situations. We also know that it can be a bit strained for parents (and occasionally for children) when they know people are watching from behind a one-way mirror. Nonetheless, we find that this part of the evaluation gives us a chance to see the kinds of behaviors that are of concern. We should also mention, however, that parent-child observations are not a standard component of most ADHD evaluations, in part because playrooms with observation suites are uncommon.

After completion of the observation phase, the child leaves with one of our assistants for further interviewing and for testing with the GDS and other appropriate psychological tests. The parents remain with a clinician to review their concerns and answer an outrageous number of questions about the child's growth history, school performance, peer and sibling relationships, and hobbies. Most of the questions we ask are designed to get a clear picture of the problems. We need to know when they started, when they tend to occur, what you do about them, what happens following attempts at discipline, and how consistent you are when it comes to disciplining your child. While you are being bombarded by questions, please keep in mind that we do not expect you to remember every date of a significant developmental milestone or to feel absolutely confident about your judgments. Nobody will think you're dull if you can't remember how old one of your six children was when he first sat up. What the clinician is most interested in is specific examples of problem behaviors and how they were handled. He or she also needs to know about birth and family history to explore the possibility that your child's problems are related in some way to heredity or to the consequence of problems at birth, such as loss of oxygen or low birth weight.

As for the day of the appointment, make sure to bring with you prior psychological reports, school records, notes from teachers, medical reports and any other written materials that might be at all relevant. Review of this information can help the clinician develop an accurate record of past efforts and opinions. In addition, it lightens reliance on your memory. We also find it useful when parents bring in some examples of the child's current school work so we can see for ourselves how routine assignments are handled. While you don't need to cart in all the potholders from first grade Art class, the more information available the better.

There's one more absolutely critical source of information that too often is unavailable to us on appointment day. This individual has daily contact with the child, is intimately involved with the family as a whole, and can represent a powerful ally in a mother's efforts to effect changes at home and school. Yes, we're talking about fathers. Roughly a third of fathers who are living within the family fail to come in for our evaluation, even though it's made clear in all our registration materials and initial phone contacts that we need their input. Fathers often have a different perspective from mothers and can add immensely to the wealth of information we need to collect.

Father's involvement is so important that all efforts should be expended to make it possible. Marital separation or divorce does not diminish the need for a father to participate in some manner. If the situation does not allow both biological parents to come together to the interview, then alternative arrangements can be made. The plea for paternal involvement certainly extends to stepfathers, so many of whom are heavily invested in the child's welfare.

While you are involved in the evaluation process, it is inevitable that you will at some point (if not constantly) wonder if the problems are not all your "fault." Even if you've decided that you're not totally to blame, you perhaps will wonder if you've handled things poorly. You should feel free to discuss issues of guilt or remorse with the clinician and try your best to gain comfort in confronting the situation. While guilt can help spur you on to making good changes, it also can get in the way if you are too caught up in it.

Parents who fail to follow up with appointments are often those who are afraid that the clinician will ultimately proclaim them failures. In reality, the clinician simply is not interested in who's to blame. We know too well that these kinds of problems are complex and never the consequence of a single individual's deeds. But we do need to understand how the various factors came together to produce difficulties so that we can suggest reasonable interventions.

After all the information is gathered, the clinician goes to work making sense of it. Depending on the practitioner and the amount of information available, you can hear at least some feedback after one or two sessions. The clinician may decide that additional assessment is necessary before arriving at a firm diagnosis. This is especially the case if he or she is suspicious of a learning problem or a severe emotional disorder. Evaluation for these kinds of problems require additional effort, often times by other professionals.

As for the feedback session itself, don't hesitate to take notes or even to tape record the interview. You will be confronted with a barrage of information and may well want the opportunity to hear it again or at least to review your notes. You should also insist on receiving a written report from the clinician that summarizes the findings. This gives you something concrete to study at your own pace and also a document that can be presented to other clinicians or to school officials.

Clinical reports need not be confusing or overly-technical. Here's an example of the sort of report we send to parents who come to our clinic. We will write more formal ones if necessary but rarely have had to do so. Again, this is our own particular style of communicating the information. Reports can be written in a sharply different format and still be useful:

Dear Mr. and Mrs. Jones:

Thank you for your recent involvement with our clinic. We are writing to review the findings of Jason's Attention Deficit Hyperactivity Disorder (ADHD) evaluation which was conducted on June 17, 1990. Our assessment is based on interviews with you and Jason, standardized behavior rating scales completed both by parents and teacher, and specialized testing for attention and self-control which we administered to Jason. Extra copies of this report are provided in order that you may share the information with other interested individuals.

Data from all sources paint a picture of a bright and charming but highly inattentive and distractible youngster who has significant difficulty coping with situations that require sustained attention or the adherence to routine rules. Despite above-average intelligence and a desire to please others, Jason finds it difficult to apply himself academically such that he is significantly underachieving and is being considered for retention next year. Problems with attention and self-control had an early onset and have been consistent throughout his development and academic history. While efforts to structure his educational and home environment have been somewhat successful, they have not helped him to the point where he is able to produce at grade level. As you know, his problems with impulsiveness and inattention are not limited to the school environment. Despite your efforts to structure his environment carefully, his poor self-control frequently gets him into trouble. It is also clear from your reports that Jason's self-esteem and mood suffer when he confronts frequent disapproval of his behavior.

In our clinic, Jason proved to be a very charming and verbal youngster with good social skills. Nevertheless, he had difficulty settling down to tasks and made attempts to distract adults from enforcing the rules at hand. His performance on standardized measures of attention and self-control documented his problems with attention, especially in distracting situations. All scores fell within an Abnormal range. He also required more structuring by the examiner than is typical.

Overall, the evidence points to a boy who experiences an Attention Deficit Hyperactivity Disorder in that he clearly meets criteria for chronicity, pervasiveness and severity. Furthermore, his problems cannot easily be accounted for by other factors such as learning disabilities or conduct problems.

As we have discussed, it will continue to be very important for both home and school to exercise the highest degree of structure possible around managing Jason's behavior. The behavior modification program that he has been involved with since last year should definitely be continued as long as necessary. It should also be reviewed frequently to make sure that it targets the appropriate problem behaviors and provides consistent and immediate consequences when he is off-task. The attached guidelines for teachers dealing with an ADHD child may be useful for them in working with Jason.

As we also discussed, I would be hesitant to retain this child given his need for an enriched academic program. My fear would be that he would become bored with repetitive material and be all the more likely to act out. It may make more sense to offer resource help geared to providing him with an opportunity to review material in a one-to-one situation. I would also suggest that the school do whatever is necessary to limit the amount of homework that he is responsible to complete after school hours. Because school is difficult enough for him to cope with in its own right, the extra hours at night may represent more of a problem than a help. We have already communicated to his school our willingness to consult with them in the future around Jason's educational needs.

Because Jason is falling significantly behind in school and is also showing some real signs of depression, a trial of medication appears warranted. It may be that a favorable response to stimulant therapy could allow for more successful and manageable behavior and academic achievement. As always, it will be very important for any medication program to be well monitored and sensibly administered. It definitely should not represent the only approach to treatment. We can be involved in that monitoring to the extent to which your physician and you desire.

Please feel free to contact us should you have any further questions or require additional information.

Sincerely,

Michael Gordon, Ph.D.
Professor of Psychiatry, Director, ADHD Clinic

We also include a profile sheet that summarizes the essential scores from rating scales and testing. This is the sheet that accompanied the report we just presented:

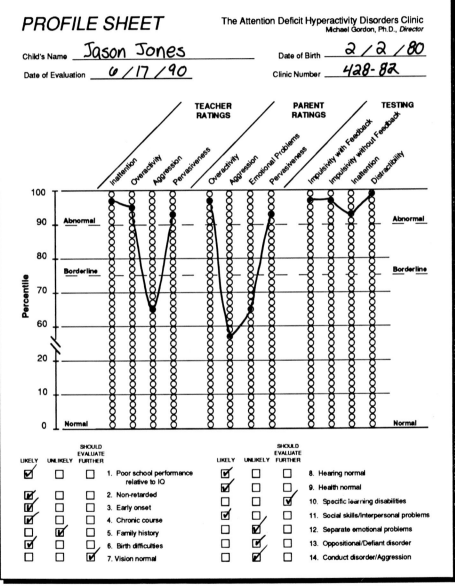

Having pleaded with you to pursue a comprehensive evaluation, we now warn you against seeking so many opinions and tests that treatment never happens (or is unnecessarily delayed). At some point, there needs to be some clear decisions regarding the nature of your child's problem and the best ways to deal with it. While there may be good reasons for getting one more opinion, make sure you are not searching for answers that are either already available or never forthcoming (such as, "Exactly why is he hyperactive?").

Finally, remember our suggestions in Critical Principle 4 about developing a close, collaborative relationship with professionals. If you don't understand some of the jargon or you feel something doesn't make sense, ASK!!!

With that bit of advice, we now move on to treatment issues.

PRINCIPLE 12

Chances Are It's Not the Lights, a Vitamin Deficiency, Sugar, or Red Dye #2

Parents and professionals desperately want to understand what causes ADHD/Hyperactivity. We all hope that there exists some clear-cut reason why hyperactive children are hyperactive. If we could find a straightforward biological explanation, the theory goes, then uncomplicated treatments would be just around the corner.

The blunt but accurate answer to the question "What causes ADHD/Hyperactivity?" is simply "We don't know." We do know it has something to do with a constitutional predisposition toward inattention and impulsiveness. In other words, many ADHD/Hyperactive children seem to arrive in the world with temperaments that leave them difficult to manage. Part of the basis for this predisposition for some children may well be heredity. It is not at all unusual for the child to be described as a "chip off the old block" or for us to hear about cousins with ADHD or grandparents who, while never officially diagnosed, had a long history of inattentive and overactive behavior.

Research on family transmission of the disorder indicates a higher likelihood that a child will exhibit symptoms associated with ADHD if one or both parents have histories that suggest the presence of similar problems. But heredity is by no means always an easy explanation because many ADHD children come from families in which there is no evidence of a precedent for these types of behavior.

Other commonly-presumed causes of ADHD symptoms are birth-related difficulties, such as low birth weight, prematurity, postmaturity, long labor, or fetal distress. Factors such as maternal drug and alcohol ingestion, smoking during pregnancy, lead poisoning, and the effects of various chemical toxins have also been considered as potential causes of ADHD. You must realize, however, that there is no way of determining if a child's ADHD/Hyperactivity is due to one particular culprit or another. Even if there were a way of establishing that the ADHD symptoms were due to low birth weight, genes, or some other biological factor, it would be unlikely that this knowledge would in any meaningful way affect decisions around treatment.

Our current understanding, then, is that this problem evolves from a conspiracy of factors which interact to form an impulsive child. Often there is this temperamentally active, unrestrained child who requires special care and structure. Unfortunately, we may find such a child in home and/or school settings that, for whatever reason, have trouble meeting the ADHD child's unique needs.

What we are most sure about is that simple explanations do not apply to the bulk of children we consider to be hyperactive. We know that fluorescent lights are not the villains, and that vitamin deficiencies play little if any role. (In fact, large doses of megavitamins can be toxic to children and there are reports of hospitalizations of children who were treated in this manner.)

The issue of diet and hyperactivity cannot be dispensed with as easily because of the staggering amount of publicity, controversy, and research that has been generated over the past 15 years. Few parents seek professional advice without first attempting to manage the problem nutritionally. The notion that food reactions are at the heart of childhood behavior problems was energetically promoted by Dr. Benjamin Feingold, an allergist. He claimed that a high percentage of children diagnosed as hyperactive were actually manifesting the effects of food allergies. Dr. Feingold suggested a rather strict elimination diet to pinpoint the troublesome foods and then a maintenance diet that restricted them. Sugar, chocolate, and various food additives were implicated as the most likely allergens.

To determine whether or not this was a valid treatment, dozens of research projects explored the impact of dietary changes on hyperactive children's behavior. For example, researchers would solicit ratings of a child's behavior from parents and teachers, feed the child huge quantities of sugar, and then obtain a second set of ratings. Typically, the child would then be rated a third time several weeks after the sugar "challenge." The resounding finding from these kinds of studies is that, at most, only 2 – 5% of hyperactive children are hyperactive primarily because of allergic reactions. This conclusion stands in stark contrast to the original claims that at least three quarters of all hyperactive children suffer from food allergies. It seems that, while some children's behavior deteriorates upon ingestion of certain foods, most children behave the same regardless of what they had for lunch or at snacktime.

The point here is that food reactions alone cannot account for the kinds of behaviors exhibited by ADHD/Hyperactive children. While all children (and adults for that matter) can become more irritable or active in reaction to certain foods, the majority of hyperactive children are still ADHD/Hyperactive on diets. The evidence against diets as a cure is strong enough now that the professional community is shying away from the entire approach. Nonetheless, there is usually no harm in monitoring your child's food intake with an eye toward changes in behavior, and restricting those foods that seem problematic. Most of those foods aren't all that healthy anyway. What we caution you against is pinning high hopes on a diet as the "ANSWER." While it may be significant for a few children, diets in most instances will be at best a small piece of the treatment puzzle. In fact, many studies indicate that the effect of diet stems more from its impact on the mother-child relationship (because it is a very structured and individualized activity) than from the diet itself.

One potential down-side of diets that we have noticed concerns the extent to which they can deprive children of the "goodies" that make life enjoyable. One of our more articulate patients complained to his mother, "It's bad enough being hyperactive, but it's worse when you're hyperactive and can't eat a Milky Way." It's true that ADHD children are less likely than others to have satisfying experiences through a school day. Maybe we're showing our own love of edibles, but it can seem unfortunate when children already limited in opportunities for enjoyment are deprived of favorite foods.

Discussion of the diet issue leads naturally to a more general principle.

PRINCIPLE 13

There Are No Magic Cures for ADHD/Hyperactivity

The hardest step for you as a parent of an ADHD/ Hyperactive child to take is in accepting that the problems will not disappear with a magic stroke. When parents of hyperactive children get together for mutual support, a recurring theme is the need to grieve and come to terms with the fact that their children suffer from a chronic problem that requires intense effort at treatment in multiple areas. In light of what we know about the disorder, the goal of treatment is to teach survival skills to both you and your child. We feel strongly that you should be wary of anybody who offers you something akin to an instant cure.

It is important that our comments not be read by you as doom and gloom predictions about a life of misery. As you will read, there are ways of dealing with hyperactivity that can lead to improvements at home and school. Moreover, the ADHD/Hyperactive child who has received the appropriate help from you, the school, and his or her doctors can adjust well and learn to cope. While it is a myth that children outgrow ADHD/Hyperactivity, it is also untrue that all ADHD children are inevitably headed for a life of poor self-control. It seems that the outcome depends to a large extent on the severity of the problem, the age at which it was diagnosed, the resources available in your child's environment, and the amount of support and encouragement you can find for yourself. Again, we aren't saying "Nothing can be done," but we are telling you that results will more likely flow from a comprehensive and long-term effort than it will from a single pill or six-week training program.

As we have indicated throughout, many therapies for ADHD have been proposed which either never have been properly studied or have been examined and found not to be of benefit. Here's a partial list of these non-remedies:

Discredited or Unproven "Cures" for ADHD

1. REMOVAL OF SUGAR OR FOOD ADDITIVES FROM THE CHILD'S DIET —We covered this topic at some length in the previous section, so we'll just reiterate that there is little evidence that dietary approaches normalize behavior for most, if not all, ADHD children. A reasonable diet never hurts and it may in fact help to keep from making matters worse, but diet alone is not the "ANSWER."

2. MEGAVITAMIN THERAPY — As you know, some health food devotees and nutritionists advocate massive ingestion of certain vitamins both for regular body maintenance as well as for the treatment of physical problems. Regimens have been proposed for the treatment of ADHD with high doses of several vitamins. To the best of our knowledge, no evidence exists to support the efficacy of this approach. In fact, a carefully-controlled study demonstrated that megavitamins were ineffective in reducing the symptoms of ADHD children. Of more concern was the fact that blood levels of vitamins were so high as to approach toxicity. Too much of anything can be dangerous.

3. EFAMOL SUPPLEMENTS — The Hyperactive Children's Support Group in England has suggested that hyperactive children suffer from a deficiency of unsaturated fatty acids which, in turn, leads to abnormally low levels of hormones called prostaglandins. They claimed that a fatty acid

supplement named Efamol, made from Oil of Evening Primrose, corrected this imbalance and led to a reduction of ADHD symptoms. A scientifically-controlled study by Dr. Eugene Arnold of The Ohio State University cast doubt on this proposal because Efamol failed to produce significant treatment effects. (We became a bit skeptical when we saw an advertisement in a health magazine for a new nail polish remover that contained Efamol.)

4.   CAFFEINE — Because caffeine is a mild stimulant that has served many of us well in improving alertness, it seemed to make sense that a cup of coffee in the morning might have some beneficial effect for the ADHD/Hyperactive child. Unfortunately, at least ten studies have shown caffeine, whether in coffee or in a tablet, to have no measurable positive impact on the inattention of an ADHD youngster. These studies have still not deterred clinicians from recommending that parents try "Juan Valdez" therapy. More often than not, this presents parents who already have enough on their hands getting Johnny out the door and on the bus, with one more morning battle. A teacher of one of our nine year old patients complained that the boy spent most of his morning running to the bathroom. She assumed this was another manifestation of his avoidance and overactivity. We learned from his mother that, at the doctor's suggestion, she poured three to four cups of coffee down his gullet every breakfast. At least we found one component of his ADHD behavior that had a clear-cut biological cause!

5.   REMOVAL OF FLUORESCENT LIGHTS — Among the more unusual propositions put forth is that behavior problems, including learning disabilities and ADHD/Hyperactivity, are caused by the untoward effects of fluorescent lighting. Proponents of this "G.E./Westinghouse" Hypothesis claimed that academic disabilities would be resolved if schools replaced fluorescent fixtures with incandescent ones. No evidence for this notion exists either.

6. SENSORY MOTOR INTEGRATION, VESTIBULAR TREATMENTS, AND COORDINATION TRAINING — Another unproven approach to the treatment of ADHD, especially popular among occupational therapists, focuses on the child's balance, coordination, and integration of multiple senses. These treatments involve either prescription of motion sickness medicine, or muscle and balance training. While the physical therapy may improve coordination, there is no data to support use of such programs for treating either ADHD or learning disabilities.

7. BIOFEEDBACK TRAINING & RELAXATION EXERCISES — While they are wholly legitimate methods for treating many physical and emotional disorders, the use of programmed feedback and relaxation has not been found helpful for ADHD children. Like many treatments that attempt to train behaviors in an office setting, whatever improvements may be achieved in training sessions tend not to generalize to daily life. More about this issue later.

What Are the Essential Elements of a Comprehensive Program for ADHD?

A comprehensive program for ADHD attacks the problem on three fronts: school, home and (if necessary) medication. Effective educational and parenting strategies must always be in force in every case, while the role of medication depends on the severity of the problem and the child's response to trials of medication. Your role as parent is to ensure as best you can that treatment efforts do not focus on just one leg of the three-part strategy. A wonderful educational plan will have limited long-term success if efforts on the home front are lagging. Conversely, well-tuned parenting skills will have less impact if the child spends most of the day in a school program that fails to provide for an ADHD youngster's basic educational needs. And, without question, medication even at mammoth doses cannot overcome the effects of poor parenting and schooling. **Medication alone is never enough!**

We will be covering important concepts involved in effective treatment along each of the treatment fronts. We'll start with medication, not because it is most important, but because it represents the most controversial and, for many parents, frightening component.

PRINCIPLE 14

For Children with Bona fide ADHD/Hyperactivity, Medication Can Truly Help — If You Do It Right

Few issues in the area of child mental health raise as much controversy and conflict as the prescription of medication for attention deficits and hyperactivity. You will find no shortage of extreme positions both for and against the use of medication. One day you might read how it is destroying our youth and the next how it represents true salvation for the ADHD youngster. The temperature of the debate has recently risen with the efforts of semi-religious groups such as the Church of Scientology's "Citizen's Committee on Human Rights." CCHR has expended considerable resources encouraging litigation and protest.

The intense controversy around medication has proven to be a mixed blessing. Professionals become frustrated because debate often falls outside of what we consider to be the realities of research and clinical experience. We also worry about legislation that can outlaw a reasonable clinical option. But it has also spawned an extraordinary amount of research and has caused both parents and clinicians to approach the administration of medications with more caution. It is far less common nowadays for a physician to say, "Try this, it might work. You can call me in 6 months and let me know."

There are literally hundreds of well-controlled research studies concerning all facets of drug response. These studies have explored issues ranging from biological mechanisms, to the effects of medication on academic functioning, to their impact on baseball playing and neighborhood popularity. While you may have strong opinions about whether or not, on principle, children should be medicated for behavior problems, you can not legitimately make a claim that stimulants (the most prevalent class of medications prescribed for ADHD/Hyperactivity) are administered without scientific foundation. Indeed, it is by far the most thoroughly investigated issue in the entire realm of medical treatments for mental health disorders of childhood.

We have no intention here of surveying the massive literature on medication response, because reviews of these studies are plentiful, current and easily available. We direct your attention particularly to the books by Drs. Barkley, Ingersoll, Goldstein, and Wender listed in the "Resources" section. Our goal is, instead, to once again help set your sights appropriately so that you can make informed and balanced decisions.

If you put passions aside and examine objectively all available evidence, it is hard not to arrive at the conclusion that stimulants, if administered properly to well-evaluated children, produce significant and meaningful improvement for approximately three-quarters of ADHD patients. Study after study employing the most careful scientific methods document the beneficial effects of stimulants in increasing attentiveness, reducing distractibility and fidgetiness, and improving overall academic and social functioning.

What Do You Actually See When a Child Takes Medication?

The child who responds to stimulants will appear calmer, less impulsive, and more able to complete tasks in an organized and planful fashion. Parents and teachers generally describe the medication responder as suddenly and unaccountably (other than for the medication) thinking about the consequences of actions, and as more able to deploy attention and effort successfully. A child who is appropriately medicated **will not** exhibit gross and alarming changes in personality or mood. Despite the sensational claims made on morning talk shows and by rabid opponents, you will not see the child transformed into a zombie or take after neighbors with pick-axes and chain saws. For that matter, he will not suddenly turn into a midget or become obsessed with suicide.

If you ask children who are on medication what it's like for them, they will generally tell you that they don't actually feel terribly different. Instead, they report finding themselves doing things (or, in some cases, not doing things) that prior to the medication would have been uncharacteristic of their behavior. Eleven year old Keith told us that he knew the medication must be "working" because his handwriting had improved markedly (not an uncommon effect of medication) and that he wasn't being yelled at by the teacher for doing annoying things like drumming on the table or chewing on pencils. While he was not at all pleased about trying the medication, he did acknowledge that he was able to finish his homework in about one third the time and that he wasn't getting into trouble with his brother as much. Actually, he was worried about coming to our clinic for another evaluation because he was concerned we would suggest termination of the medication.

In our clinical experience, response to medication falls into three general categories. First is the "DRA-MATIC, NO DOUBT ABOUT IT, PRAISE THE LORD" response, which tends to make us look brilliant. Children who fall into this category show remarkable changes in their behavior that cannot plausibly be attributed to anything other than the impact of the medication. These are the youngsters who go from F's to A's in one marking period, suddenly are able to carry on lengthy and thoughtful conversations with astonished parents, or sit through a meal without incident. One parent of a dramatic responder talked in terms of the "war zone" of her household being demobilized, while another was shocked that her previously out-of-control five year old would sit on her lap for 30 minutes to listen to a story. For children in the Dramatic category, the medication seems to significantly thin that unusually thick barrier we talked about earlier. Suddenly, the child tunes into meaningful cues within the environment and is able to be appropriately guided by normal rewards, punishments and incentives.

The next general category of responders is the, "IT SEEMS TO HELP" group. While parents and teachers notice improvement in the child's attention and self-control, the effects are not of the astonishing variety. A teacher might tell us, "He's definitely easier to teach because he's not quite so fidgety and distractible, but he still requires a ton of extra attention. The medication definitely seems to help but it sure doesn't put him at the head of the class." Most children fall into this category of medication response. There are significant improvements but not wholesale changes that instantaneously produce bliss.

One phenomenon we have learned to look for occurs when parents report a modest or nonexistent medication response based on their observations of the child's behavior in the evening or on weekends when no medication had been administered. Many times parents tell us that they stopped medication because they couldn't see any differences for themselves, even though the teacher did tell them that school performance had improved. Never forget that the most popular and effective stimulants, Ritalin and Dexedrine, are short-acting medications. They tend to be at their most potent about an hour after ingestion and are typically ineffective by the third or fourth hour. Consequently, if your child's last dose is at noon, you will not see any medication effects at six or seven o'clock at night. Most of the benefits of stimulants are obvious only while the medication is active. If you give your child a dose when he awakens at 6:30 a.m., don't expect significant improvement in an 11 o'clock math class. By that point, the medication has been broken down by the body and is no longer effective. You have to experiment with doses and schedules that best match demands for attention and self-control.

The short-acting nature of Ritalin and Dexedrine is a mixed blessing. On the one hand, their quick action makes it easy to observe medication effects and adjust the dosage. You don't need to build up the medication in the bloodstream over several weeks or even wait hours to observe changes. You can give a youngster the dose and observe effects in as little as one-half hour. There also are no withdrawal effects with Ritalin or Dexedrine; anytime you want to stop them to compare how the child behaves off medication, you can do so safely. If a child develops serious side effects to the extent that medication needs to be halted, they almost invariably disappear as the medication becomes inactive. The short active life of the medication is likely also the reason why there are no reports of long-term health effects of stimulant therapy. The chemicals do not seem to hang around the body long enough to cause ongoing physical harm.

While there are many benefits to a short-acting medication, there are also prices to be paid. It's bothersome to parents, school and child to have the up-and-down effects of stimulants rather than an even and consistent benefit. Arrangements need to be made with the school nurse to administer a late-morning and/or afternoon dose. Moreover, the child isn't always thrilled about having to leave the classroom to receive the medication. This is especially the case for adolescents who already might have experienced discomfiture with the need for medication. You will read shortly how pharmaceutical manufacturers have attempted and failed to formulate a longer acting stimulant with the same benefits as the short-acting variety.

The last category of medication response is "THE STUFF'S NO GOOD OR NOT WORTH IT" type. Some children either don't respond or react poorly to medication for reasons that are not always clear. Despite all efforts to find the right medication at the right dose we have had situations in which positive medication response has absolutely eluded us. At other times medication has all the desired impact on attention and self-control but also causes troublesome side effects that make the medication "not worth it."

Obviously, if medications don't work or are more trouble than they are worth, don't use them. The only caution we have is that you not jump ship before you pursue this option fully. Too often parents and clinicians will give up if a single dosage of a single medication has limited or untoward consequences. These medications can work in mysterious ways and you risk overlooking benefit by abandoning a trial hastily. This lesson was forcefully driven home to us several years ago when we were involved in the monitoring of a medication trial for seven year-old Danny. At 5 milligrams of Ritalin, Danny was by all accounts worse (which took some doing because he was generally uncontrollable). His mother told us that he was literally bouncing off the walls and acting oddly. At the next higher dose of 10 milligrams, his behavior became strikingly normal. Persistence with the trial had clear payoff for this child.

If you're going to take the leap to medication, do it right. Work with a physician who is thoroughly knowledgeable about medication options and will work closely with you in a sophisticated and responsive manner. Most of the horror stories about Ritalin, at least those that have a basis in reality, stem from improper diagnosis and from clinicians not making sure that medications are properly evaluated and monitored.

As you can gather, we see medication as a reasonable treatment option for children who are appropriately evaluated and when medications are handled by knowledgeable clinicians who take the time to monitor them carefully and are both willing and able to adjust dosages and drugs to insure optimal response. You certainly have noticed all the qualifications of our support for this option. Medication for ADHD children can help but only if you approach it reasonably. And, as you have heard, only if other components of the treatment program are in place.

Despite our acknowledgement of the potential benefits of medication, you should never feel bullied by school, physician, or anyone else into trying the medication until you have become completely informed and feel comfortable with the diagnosis, comprehensiveness of the overall treatment program, and the physician's style. While the stimulants are safe as far as medications are concerned, they are still drugs and should not be taken lightly (in any sense of the phrase). While you shouldn't automatically dismiss medication as an option, you should also not feel pressured into a quick decision.

How Do I Decide Whether or Not To Try Medication?

Of the many questions we've asked for you over these pages, this is perhaps the hardest to answer in such a way that it addresses your personal situation. Some calls are easier to make than others. We feel most comfortable recommending medication when children are so impulsive that they are at risk for (or actually have) hurt themselves or others. A five year old we evaluated had been in the emergency room six times in two years for one injury or another, all of which stemmed from his complete obliviousness to the consequences of his actions. He had also started a fire in the garage during the two minutes his mother went inside to answer the phone. Despite his youth, we felt that his pervasive disinhibition warranted a trial of medication.

The other conditions that make the medication decision more straightforward are when serious non-medical treatment options are knocking at the door. Before 11 year-old Stan, who has an IQ of 128, was placed in a self-contained classroom for severely Learning Disabled children because of his persistent inattention and underachievement, his parents decided to try medication. While they had longstanding reservations about the use of stimulants, they were also aware of the potential "side effects" of special class placement for Stan. They felt that medication might help Stan attend well enough to maintain a regular class placement. Fortunately, Stan was a "Dramatic" responder who managed one of the more impressive academic turn-arounds in his school's history.

What are some other guidelines for the medication decision? If you have fully implemented tailored programs at home and school and your child still isn't succeeding, then medication may make sense. Or, if implementation of these programs is impossible because he or she can't sit or attend long enough to even orient to the program, then, again, medication may be a reasonable option.

Another tipoff is when the child's self-esteem is so battered by failure and by the struggle to maintain control that signs of depression surface. ADHD youngsters, especially those who are eager to please, are not immune to the impact of chronic frustration. One teenager told us, "There's no way I can be like the other kids in class, so what's the point? I'd rather just stay home and sleep or watch TV." When a youngster becomes despairing of his circumstance and feels that there is no salvation from the consequences of his impulsiveness and inattention, a trial of medication may be warranted.

Professional opinions vary on when to initiate a trial of medication. Some clinicians feel that the medicine should be tried immediately, at the same time other aspects of a comprehensive program are developed. The rationale for this approach is that precious time and opportunities for helping to set the child on a normal developmental course can be lost while exploring other options. Why wait to try a relatively safe medication, the argument goes, that may have major impact on the child's ability to succeed? This style of clinical management is not without merit. However, except in extreme cases of the sort mentioned above or when timing becomes a critical factor (e.g., the school year is almost over and you want teachers familiar with your child's behavior to be involved in a drug trial), we tend to take a more step-wise approach. We like to see parents and schools try other strategies before launching into medication. In this way we can be assured that non-medical programs alone are insufficient to bring about improvements. A conservative starting point also keeps all involved from relying solely on the medication. We want to avoid the "We don't have to do anything 'cause he's on Ritalin" mentality that can too frequently rear its ugly head. We have also found that parents are more comfortable with trying the medication if they know that other avenues have first been explored.

Your comfort level regarding the medication is no small matter for successful drug treatment. Parents who are at ease with their decision are much more likely to adhere to administration schedules and deal with the many issues that can arise during the course of treatment. We are ever-mindful of the fact that roughly 40% of children placed on medication, even when they respond positively, are not still on that medication four months later. Our experience is that effective management of the medication requires a commitment on the part of the family to give it a fair shot.

Your child must also be informed and at ease about the medication if you want any chance at an enduring medication response. Like most things in life, it's not so much what you do but how you do it that spells the difference between success and failure. If your child hears you say, "You need to take your medicine because you're always bad and this pill will make you good," or a teacher say to the class, "Johnny's terrible behavior shows us that he obviously didn't get his medicine to-day," he will undoubtedly develop negative feelings about taking medication. No one wants to hear that their goodness or badness depends on a little pill or that acceptance by others is completely tied to medication. Children taking medication need to know that it is intended not as a replacement for their personal responsibility but as an aide in helping them pay better attention and think a bit more carefully before they act. We like youngsters to understand that the medicine is designed to help them deal with a legitimate problem that they have paying attention. We also are intent on communicating that being on medication in no way relieves them of stewardship over their actions. Clearly, the manner in which this attitude is communicated depends very much on the child's age and abilities, not to mention your willingness to listen and respond to his or her concerns. You should find your clinician ready and able to talk with your child about the medication and answer his questions.

You will notice that we've addressed our comments largely to the process of deciding whether or not to **try** the medication. What you should be thinking about is the worthwhileness of a medication trial and not necessarily about a commitment to medication forever. You need to enter this arena with the mind set of an experimenter who is intent on exploring the usefulness of medication. Fortunately, as we discussed above, there are not many risks inherent in this experiment if you and your clinician work together collaboratively.

Why do some children not respond as dramatically (or at all)? We don't know exactly. It seems tied to severity of the problem and also to the extent to which other problems complicate the situation. In other words, children who are ADHD/Hyperactive but also learning disabled, aggressive, anxious, or emotionally disturbed will tend to respond less dramatically. This now brings us to our next critical principle.

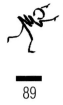

PRINCIPLE 15

Medication Is Not One Size Fits All

We'll take an opportunity here to expand on the concept we most fervently want to convey regarding medication. Children have remarkably individualized reactions to the various medications used to treat ADHD/ Hyperactivity. It always astounds us how the same dose of a stimulant, administered to ten children of similar age, weight and problem severity, can have ten unique results. One child may respond dramatically without side effects, another might become mildly depressed, yet another might have a positive response but become completely uninterested in eating lunch. It's one thing for us to talk about how children generally respond to medication, but quite another to find out how your particular child will fare. What would be your child's response to medication? You really don't know until a trial is initiated. And that brings us to the next question:

How Do You Go About a Reasonable Trial of Medication?

We'll start by describing to you the "Sears Best" approach to medication trials. This top-of-the-line strategy, usually (but not always) conducted in university settings, involves what's called a double-blind, multiple dose, placebo protocol. Sounds complicated but it's actually more time consuming than elaborate. Over a several-week period, your child is administered either a low dose, a higher dose, or placebo (a sugar pill that looks the same as the active medication). The order in which the different dose levels are tried is chosen randomly and no one except for a nurse or technician knows which phase of the trial is which (this is the "blind" part). The reason for the blind trial is to prevent opinions about the impact of the medication from being influenced by the knowledge that the youngster is on medication at a particular dose. Someone who has advocated pharmacotherapy (treatment with medication) may unconsciously overstate positive drug effects as a way of supporting his or her position. Conversely, a parent or teacher who adamantly opposes medication may subtly or otherwise minimize improvements in the child's behavior. Human judgments are, by their nature, frail and much at the mercy of forces from within and without the observer. A blind trial is one scientific technique for controlling such influences.

At the end of each week of the trial, the parents and teachers are asked to complete the same set of rating scales that were administered as part of the initial evaluation. In this way, the clinician can track changes in the child's behavior from baseline (the child's typical behavior before treatment) at various doses and with the placebo. At the end of each week the child is also brought back for re-testing on laboratory measures such as the Gordon Diagnostic System and for assessment of side effects. At the end of the third week, the code is broken and the clinician learns which weeks were associated with which dose. He can then chart the ratings and test scores over the course of the trial and determine which dose, if any, produced optimal effects. It may turn out, for example, that teacher ratings and test scores improved most significantly at the higher dose but that unacceptable side effects were present at that level. Or it may be that low doses produced no effects on classroom behavior but caused major improvement according to the parents. The point is that this kind of systematic trial allows us all to see for ourselves how the medication works.

How about the child who does as well or better on the placebo pill? Clearly, the expectation is that behavior should revert to baseline levels while the child is taking a pill that has no pharmacological action. Nonetheless, roughly 25% of children studied in this sort of careful drug protocol show a placebo response. It's fascinating that this percentage of improvement during a placebo phase is generally the same when any psychiatric medication is studied. It just seems to be a quality of human nature that believing you're getting help is helpful even when you're not really getting it. With ADHD children, it may also be that part of the placebo response is related to how adults rate children differently when medication effects are being evaluated. In other words, those influences on perception we talked about above may alter someone's sensitivity to positive changes in behavior. We have also found that placebo effects with ADHD children are short-lived. It doesn't take too long for the power of positive thinking to diminish when demands for attention and self-control persist.

While the "Sears Best" approach to medication trials is the most scientific and informative strategy, it is not always practical for either parent or clinician. Even getting the placebo pills can be a challenge because they have to be ordered from the manufacturer so that they look like the active medication. Monitoring of medication can fall short of the double-blind, placebo trial and still be meaningful. At the least, the rating scales and testing should be readministered after a week or two of trial. This boils down to asking the teacher to fill out the forms and then call you (and/or the clinician) after your child's been on the medication a suitable period of time.

In this way you will at least have some documentation of the impact the medication has on your child's behavior. What you want to avoid is placing your son or daughter on medication and never having any professional monitoring of the drug effects. At the risk of redundancy, we will restate that it is absolutely imperative that your physician be directly involved in contacting the school and in touching base with you over the course of the trial.

Even when your child has been on medication for months or years, you can always reinitiate a trial at different doses or go off the medicine entirely. As children grow, they often require somewhat more medicine to achieve the same level of benefit. (Actually, it's sometimes unclear whether higher doses are a consequence of physical changes or the steady increase in demands for attention as the grade levels are climbed.) You might also start wondering if the medicine is still necessary. No harm will befall your child by withdrawing the Ritalin or Dexedrine and seeing how he or she manages. These off-medication trials can happen accidentally if you forget to give your child a pill one morning or you haven't gotten the prescription refilled. It can be embarrassing but somewhat reassuring when the teacher calls that night and says, "Mrs. Smith, do us all a favor and don't forget his pill tomorrow morning."

How Do You Know Exactly What Dose To Give?

There are no hard and fast rules for deciding on a starting dose for the stimulants. As you've been reading, children have unique responses to these medications which are determined by age, weight, severity of the problem, and physical status. Three methods are commonly employed for establishing trial doses. The

"Standard Dose" method simply starts the child out at the lowest possible dose (5 milligrams for Ritalin and Dexedrine) and works upward until a drug response is documented. The "Weight Method" is the most popular approach to arriving at an initial dose level. The physician calculates a certain number of milligrams of medication per kilogram (2.2 pounds) of body weight. A typical low dose of Ritalin, for example, would be .3 milligrams per kilogram of body weight (or .136 milligrams of medication per pound). If a child weighs 18.2 kilograms (or 40 pounds), then the low dose would be .3 times 18.2 (or 40 times .136), all of which comes out to about 5 milligrams of Ritalin. Keep in mind that these calculations are intended as rough estimations of a good starting point. Also, the formula is used to decide on a dose **per administration** (as opposed to the total amount administered in one day). The daily dose may range anywhere from 10 milligrams up to 120 milligrams per day.

What Do I Tell the School About the Medication?

Parents are often reticent to tell the school that their child is on medication. They don't want teachers to treat him differently because of the medication or they want to "blind" the teacher to the presence or absence of medication so that an unbiased opinion can be rendered. Parents are most opposed to the school being informed when there has been unpleasantness within their relationship with school officials. The school, on the other hand, gets upset about being left in the dark about this important aspect of the student's life. "How can we deal with this problem if we're out of the loop on such a critical part of his treatment? We need to know if changes in his classroom functioning are related to our programming or to pharmacotherapy." Educators become particularly agitated when they see what looks to them like side effects but they aren't even sure if the child's on medication and aren't asked for input.

Our opinion is that the school should be informed that you will be trying your son or daughter on medication and that you will be asking the teachers to provide feedback on a regular basis regarding classroom behavior and academic achievement to help determine the medication's effectiveness. You should explain to the school that you will be enlisting their help in making decisions but that appropriate monitoring procedures are such that they may not always know, at least at the outset, exactly what protocol is being employed. You should also make it clear that you need to hear from them immediately if they notice any alarming behaviors such as twitches or social withdrawal. Finally, you need to convey to the school an attitude that shows investment in exploring and perhaps ultimately using the medication, but not to the exclusion of whatever other special educational services are warranted.

How About Afternoons, Weekends and Vacations?

The traditional approach to medication has been to limit administrations of stimulants to morning and afternoon doses during the school week. In this way the child could benefit from medication during school hours and then be free of medicine at other times. Some moderately impaired children are indeed able to manage sufficiently well outside of school grounds such that afternoon or weekend doses are unnecessary. For most children, however, the symptoms of ADHD do not suddenly disappear with the striking of the 2:30 dismissal

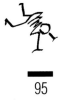
bell. There's still homework, practicing piano, chores, shopping at the mall, religious instruction, Little League, getting along with younger brother and kids in the neighborhood, dinner time, Cub Scouts, and Aunt Jane coming to visit with her three children and new puppy. All these activities are important in a child's life and certainly require considerable impulse control and attention. To our way of thinking, if a child is so severely ADHD that he requires medication, then he will likely require it on a dose schedule that spans beyond just school hours. The settling effects of medicine may allow for more successful family and peer relationships which, in turn, can lead to improved social skills and self-esteem. For this reason, it is becoming more common for physicians to prescribe three doses per day (with the afternoon dose often the smallest), seven days per week.

Decisions around medication during summer vacations are somewhat more dependent on the activities planned. Many ADHD children do relatively well if allowed to run around outside for hours at a time. They may not need medication, then, if summer days are filled mostly with bike riding and swimming. It may be a different story for the child enrolled in summer school or camp, or for the family intent on taking a cross country car trip. Why have Johnny bouncing off the walls of the Winnebago from New York to California when he, not to mention his family, would benefit much more from the experience if he could sit still and maintain some degree of control over his behavior? The importance for a child's development of joyful family times and positive out-of-school experiences should never be underestimated.

There's one more reason why we favor every-day administration of the medication for most children. We've noticed that children who take stimulants only during the day develop a two-sided sense of themselves —"Me On" and "Me Off" medicine. "While I'm on medicine I can think about what I'm doing and things don't happen so fast. When I'm off the medicine, I'm always running around and in trouble. I like the 'Me' on medicine, but that's just in school." We feel that children should, as much as possible, develop a coherent sense of them-selves and their behavior. They need to have a consis-tent feeling for how they react to their environment and how they handle matters internally. Constant changes in their sense of control and ability to reflect on situations may work against development of a more stable self-image.

A small percentage of children on medication need to be off when possible in order to gain back weight that is lost as a consequence of the pharmacotherapy. In these cases, drug holidays are reasonable strategies for dealing with one of the more common side effects.

Will He Have To Be on Medication Forever?

Once upon a time professionals told parents that children needed to take the medication only until puber-ty when, according to the prevailing theory, symptoms of hyperactivity would melt away. It was thought that the increased release of hormones during this period affect-ed brain chemistry in such a way as to correct imbalanc-es underlying the disorder. Because of careful research into the life history of individuals diagnosed as hyperac-tive in childhood, we now relegate to the status of myth the "In Come the Hormones, Out Goes the Hyperactivi-ty" theory. For most children, one or more of the primary characteristics of the disorder persists into at least early adulthood. While ADHD teenagers are not necessarily as overactive as they once were, they are often still sig-nificantly inattentive and impulsive. Vulnerabilities to academic underachievement and social maladjustment endure. As a consequence, many children, especially those who are seriously impaired, will benefit from on-going administration of medication. Within the past few years it has become more common for physicians to maintain ADHD individuals on medication on a permanent basis. This practice can be justified not only by solid evidence of ADHD as a potentially persistent handicap, but also by the lack of any indication that ADHD necessarily impairs pubertal processes, growth, or general physical health.

Although it makes no sense to keep children on medication when it no longer provides benefit, premature termination of pharmacotherapy can also lead to problems. We saw a sixteen year-old boy who had been diagnosed as hyperactive at the age of six and placed on Ritalin the following year. He had a favorable response to the medication and stayed at grade level throughout the primary grades. When the boy was twelve, the pediatrician told the parents that medication was no longer necessary or desirable now that their son was entering puberty. The next four years were marked by consistent academic failure brought about by his distractibility, inattention, and intense frustration with himself. At the time of our appointment, he had decided to drop out of school and, according to him, "give up the struggle."

Following our evaluation, we recommended that the family re-initiate a trial of medication to see if it might help him deal with school demands. Relatively low doses of medication had a striking effect on his capacity to finish tasks. We recently learned that he had graduated from high school and went on to enroll in a local community college.

PRINCIPLE 16

Know the Side Effects!!

Sensational stories aside, Ritalin and Dexedrine are generally safe medications which cause few serious side effects in the majority of children. But they nevertheless are medications and you need to be aware of problems that can arise. The most typical side effects, insomnia and loss of appetite, tend to dissipate after two to four weeks. As you might gather, whether or not your child would develop side effects depends on his or her physical makeup and reaction to these medications. What's somewhat comforting is that, even should more serious side effects develop, they tend to subside when the medicine is stopped.

By this point you probably have figured out that, if there's a definitive study in the area of ADHD, Dr. Russell Barkley has probably been involved. Such is the case with the careful exploration of side effects. Dr. Barkley and his team studied 82 children between 5 and 16 years of age who underwent a double-blind, placebo-controlled investigation of two doses of Ritalin (.3 and .5 milligrams per kilogram twice daily). The table below shows the percentage of side effects noted during the course of the trial. The most common side effects, as we noted above, were decreased appetite and insomnia as well as stomach aches and headaches. They were all rated as mild (an average of 3 out of a high ranking of 9).

TABLE 1

Percentage of 82 ADHD Children Experiencing Each Side Effect of Ritalin at Two Dose Levels (.3 and .5 mg/kg twice daily)

Possible Side Effect	Placebo		Low Dose		Mod. Dose	
	%	Sev.	%	Sev.	%	Sev.
Decreased Appetite	≤15	0.4	52	1.8	56	2.6
Insomnia	40	1.5	62	2.7	68	3.1
Stomach Aches	18	0.5	39	1.0	35	1.5
Headaches	11	0.3	26	0.6	21	0.8
Prone to Crying	49	1.8	59	2.3	54	2.0
Tics/Nervous Movements	18	0.7	18	0.9	28	1.2
Nail biting	22	1.1	26	1.1	29	1.3
Talks Excessively	16	0.4	20	0.6	22	0.9
Irritable	72	3.2	65	2.6	66	2.7
Sadness	43	1.6	48	1.9	41	1.8
Stares Excessively	40	1.3	38	1.2	38	1.0

Sev. = Mean Severity Rating of this side effect using a scale from 0 (not at all) to 9 (severe). Table reproduced with permission of Russell A. Barkley, Ph.D.

Most noteworthy is the number of side effects that appeared when the child wasn't on any medication at all (that is, during the placebo phase). You'll see that children were rated as sad, irritable, staring and talking excessively as much off the medication as while they were taking it. This tells us that unless a careful study is made of the child's typical behavior off-medication, then those same behaviors can be erroneously attributed to medication.

This study also provides additional information about medication response which highlights some of our prior discussion. Out of the 82 children, 13 percent were found to be poor- or non-responders to either dose of medication. The rest of the children showed improvements at school and home sufficient to warrant recommendations that the Ritalin be continued. Dr. Barkley also points out that, contrary to claims of the Church of Scientology, no children attempted suicide, committed murder, developed seizures or brain damage, became addicted or permanently emotionally disturbed from the medication, or developed Tourette's syndrome (more about this in a minute). However, 10 percent of the children developed mild nervous tics or nervous mannerisms at the moderate dose which subsided when medication was discontinued. One child developed mild psychotic symptoms at the moderate dose of medication which subsided within a few hours after immediately discontinuing medication.

The amount of weight lost by children for whom this side effect fails to subside typically does not reach levels that are of medical consequence. Nonetheless, your physician should keep a careful watch on the child's weight. You can minimize weight loss by being flexible about letting your child eat after mealtimes. You may find that he picks at dinner (especially if he had an afternoon dose) and then starts foraging for snacks before bedtime. You should let him eat as much as he likes after meals as a way of ensuring sufficient food intake.

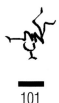

A common issue with the use of Ritalin concerns potential effects on growth. In 1972 a report appeared claiming that long-term use of Ritalin decreased height and weight at adulthood. This concern generated extensive study of growth patterns of ADHD children both on and off medication. The conclusion of these studies, according to a panel appointed by the Food and Drug Administration, is that the effects of Ritalin on adult height and weight are minimal. It turns out that there may be some suppression of growth during the first year or two of stimulant therapy, but that this phenomenon subsides by about the third year of treatment.

Another flashpoint has been the potential relationship between the use of Ritalin and development of an irreversible neurological disorder called Tourette's Syndrome. This is a condition which is characterized by involuntary motor and vocal tics. As you just read in our discussion of Dr. Barkley's study on side effects, some children can develop tics at higher doses of Ritalin which subside once the medication is discontinued. These tics are **not** associated with Tourette's Syndrome because they are reversible. However, for some children the tics persist as part of a full-blown manifestation of Tourette's.

It was once thought that Ritalin could cause Tourette's, but more recent evidence tends to point to the opposite conclusion. It happens that between 50 and 70 percent of children with Tourette's also have ADHD, and that the ADHD symptoms can precede the onset of tics by months or years. Consequently, a child who would develop Tourette's syndrome (and develop tics regardless of other treatments), might first be treated for ADHD because those are the symptoms that are first to appear. As a result of these findings, there is much less concern about this potentially serious side effect although, as you've heard from us repeatedly, you never know ahead of time the effects a medication will have on any one individual.

As for insomnia, this usually entails a child falling asleep about one hour later than typical, rather than a disrupted or fitful sleep. Usually, sleep problems can be managed by adjusting the times that doses are administered. There are occasional trade-offs between the benefits of an afternoon dose for getting homework and meals completed, and the disadvantages of children still awake when you could use a few night-time hours of serenity.

A potential side effect which can occur in children who have been on medication over many months is increased suspiciousness or paranoia. Our colleague, Dr. Martin Irwin of the SUNY Health Science Center at Syracuse, reports that this side effect is frequently overlooked and should be monitored. If you notice that your child is becoming uncharacteristically suspicious, call your physician and report this symptom.

There is no evidence that the stimulants lead to drug addiction or dependence. Children may come to rely on the medication to help them cope, but they do not exhibit physiological addiction as one might to nicotine or Valium. Remember that the stimulants don't produce a "high" in children for which they might hunger. Children can develop some tolerance to the medication within the first year or so of administration. This can be managed by increasing the dose until therapeutic effects re-appear. It is unusual that the dose would have to be increased again except as the child grows older and heavier.

Both Ritalin and Dexedrine come in longer acting versions which were developed in order to cut down on the number of doses necessary during the day. The Sustained Release formulation of Ritalin (known as Ritalin

SR) was designed to last for approximately 8 hours and keep the medication at a steady state. Unfortunately, this has not been a successful alternative for most children because it delivers too little medication at any one time. Physicians find themselves "boosting" the Ritalin SR with additional doses of the standard formulations. In our experience, it is preferable to stick with the regular medication for most cases. The same can be said of the longer-acting Dexedrine spansule which is also designed to release the medication over a longer period of time. While we have had better luck with the Dexedrine spansule than with Ritalin SR, we still find ourselves resorting more often than not to the short-acting versions.

Are There Alternatives to Stimulant Medications?

Non-stimulant medications are available for children who do not tolerate or benefit from stimulants, or have pre-existing medical conditions that preclude their use. From our point of view, these other alternative medications should be explored only with good reason and not as a first line of action. You need to keep in mind that there is relatively little known about them, despite their relatively widespread use. The hundreds of studies of Ritalin and Dexedrine stand alongside perhaps two dozen scientific studies of non-stimulants. As such, they should be approached with even greater caution than Ritalin and Dexedrine.

The leading non-stimulant alternative is a medication called imipramine (Tofranil is the product name). Despite the fact that it's what is called a tricyclic antidepressant, it has similar effects on ADHD symptoms as stimulants with the added benefits of having a more consistent action during the course of a day and of improving mood. In other words, imipramine does not have the ups and downs of effectiveness so characteristic of the stimulants. Side effects include drowsiness, dryness of mouth, blurred vision, rapid heart beat, constipation, and dizziness. These side effects are usually reversible or easily tolerated. The disadvantages of imipramine are that it is slow in taking effect and that many children develop tolerance to the medication after several months and no longer are helped. The other major downside is that, unlike stimulants, imipramine is a potentially toxic drug at levels that are too high. This medication must be monitored with blood tests and electrocardiograms on a regular basis. Our impression is that many parents are not informed fully about the potential risks involved with this medication. While we consider imipramine as a reasonable alternative for children who develop serious side effects from stimulants, you will need to become even more vigilant about health effects.

Perhaps to drive home this point, we should mention a recent report warning about the use of a tricyclic antidepressant called desipramine, which is similar to imipramine in chemical structure and is also prescribed for ADHD/Hyperactivity. According to this report, three deaths were attributed to desipramine administration in children whose blood levels of the drug were within "safe" levels. If your child is on this medication, you will certainly want to check with your physician.

A host of other medications have been prescribed for children with ADHD/Hyperactivity. They include antipsychotics (such as Haldol, Thorazine, and Mellaril), lithium, anticonvulsants (such as Tegretol), and antihypertensive medications (such as Clonidine). While there may be individual cases in which use of these medications is indicated, they generally are second or third lines of defense rather than primary options.

PRINCIPLE 17

Effective Educational Programming Starts With Acceptance of ADHD as a Legitimate Disorder That Warrants Special Handling

For an educational treatment program to fly, all aboard must first be knowledgeable about the nature of ADHD and accept its legitimacy as a *bona fide* disorder. No amount of educational techniques, tips for teachers, or lists of educational options can overcome the attitude that ADHD children are just "irresponsible," "lazy," "immature" or "spoiled."

Unless the teacher believes that your child's diagnosis is well-founded and real, it will be hard for you to convince him or her to make all the modifications necessary for effective educational management. If you are a teacher and don't understand that this child's handicap makes it nearly impossible for him to get organized, you will assume that he just does not care and you will bristle at suggestions that you should spend extra time and effort helping him to compensate. "Why should I allow him extra time to complete assignments? He's smart enough to do them if he only put forth the effort," the unconvinced teacher will surely ask. We have all too often heard teachers and administrators refuse to make alterations in a child's programming because they either were unsure of the legitimacy of the diagnosis for a particular child or were unfamiliar with the essential characteristics of the problem. They did not understand that asking the ADHD child to work diligently and efficiently for four or five hours a day is tantamount to asking the blind to see, the deaf to hear, and the lame to run.

Despite the surge of research and interest in the field of ADHD, general awareness of its existence and nature has only begun to take hold. Most school officials have only a dim conception of the disorder and usually are unfamiliar with the degree of complexity and effort involved in helping these children. To be fair, academicians have generally done a poor job translating their knowledge to those most involved with the education of ADHD/Hyperactive children on a daily basis. Any teacher will tell you that information about the disorder is hard to find and that she certainly never learned about it through the course of her education.

Unless a school has taken a special interest in learning about ADHD by sponsoring inservice training sessions and working with ADHD parent support groups, they likely have not yet educated themselves about appropriate management. Parents of the ADHD child often have to educate the educators about the problem by providing written materials, bringing in speakers to address teacher meetings, and ensuring that a child's clinician spends the time to determine that all involved are up to speed on the essential elements of a good educational program.

Acceptance of ADHD as a true and honest diagnosis is hampered by the fact that educational laws currently do not yet recognize it as a handicapping condition requiring special educational services. Public Law 94-142, which mandates provision of special services for all children who require them, does not now list ADHD as one of the handicaps that allow for eligibility. Therefore, many schools can say, "We're sorry, but ADHD is not a legal designation so we cannot provide any special services and don't need to spend time learning about the disorder."

The only way services can be offered legally is if the ADHD child can be classified under one of the identified categories, such as Learning Disabled, Emotionally Disturbed, or Other Health Impaired. However, most ADHD children do not show the kinds of discrepancies between intellectual potential and academic achievement necessary to qualify for the Learning Disabled label, and designating an ADHD child as Emotionally Disturbed also strains the bounds of credibility. At the time of this writing, intense efforts are underway to have ADHD included as a handicapping condition under the revision of Public Law 94-142. If all goes well, this most prevalent of educational problems will legally qualify for special services in the near future.

Successful implementation of an educational program also requires that everyone understand that the **typical classroom is a terrible place for an ADHD child**. If the President were to appoint a commission to design Hell for the ADHD youngster, the final plans would resemble the kinds of classrooms and curricula present in most of our schools. After all, we are asking children who have profound problems attending, organizing, and controlling their actions to spend hours per day attending, organizing, and controlling their actions. Let's not forget the essential needs of an ADHD child:

The Essential Needs of an ADHD Child

1. Clearly specified rules, expectations and instructions

2. Frequent, immediate, and consistent feedback on behavior and redirection to task

3. Reasonable and meaningful consequences for both compliance and non-compliance

4. Programming and adult intervention designed to compensate for the child's distractibility, limited organizational skills, and low frustration tolerance

5. A well-integrated and functioning team of parents, teachers, administrators and clinicians who communicate often and work together to create a structured and supportive environment

To penetrate the ADHD child's "thick barrier," his world has to provide him with unusual amounts of structure and flexibility. As we all know, a regular classroom, even in the best of times, is limited in the extent to which these needs can be addressed. In a context which places a premium on self-control and sustained attention, consequences tend to be inconsistent, infrequent and delayed. For children who are drawn to events that are most stimulating and intriguing, it is usually the case that their work is less interesting than the panorama of student activity that buzzes about a classroom. It's a lot more fun to watch another child get scolded or underground notes being passed around than to complete a sheet of math problems.

If you're an ADHD child, you'll impulsively grab for attention however it may come your way. In a classroom, the chances are far greater that you'll get attention for doing something wrong than for doing something right. ADHD youngsters are so used to being in trouble that they become accustomed to attracting a teacher's attention by negative routes rather than through compliance. And don't forget that teachers, more often than not, will have limited (if any) training in working with ADHD children and perhaps equally limited support from the administration and outside clinicians to help them develop successful strategies. Finally, opportunities to communicate with parents and others involved in the child's treatment are often on a catch-as-catch-can basis and not geared toward integrative problem solving.

All these factors conspire to create a learning environment which is hostile territory for most children with ADHD/Hyperactivity. If a child is to benefit from help, there has to be acceptance on all fronts of the incontrovertible fact that there need to be changes in standard programming to allow for some chance at survival.

PRINCIPLE 18

Educational Strategies Will Be Effective Only If the Setting Allows for Their Implementation

As you know by now, we see the ADHD youngster as bound to fail unless reasonable modifications in educational programming are instituted. If a child functions well within a regular mainstream classroom without any services, medication, or adjustments in instructional approach then, from our point of view, he's probably not all that ADHD. The question becomes, "But what kind of services?" You will hear a spectrum of opinion on the optimal learning environment for ADHD children. Some experts feel strongly that all ADHD children can be mainstreamed if supported by careful programming, teacher aides, and tailored materials. Others advocate specially-designed ADHD classrooms that are self-contained and staffed with teachers who have received specific training in this area.

Our approach is to take cues on program design from the child's individual status and from the options available. As you have heard from us, *ad nauseam,* we have not found the STANDARD ADHD CHILD on display next to the STANDARD INCH or STANDARD POUND at the Bureau of Standards in Washington. Some children's symptoms are not so severe that they cannot be maintained in a regular classroom with appropriate modifications in their program. Other youngsters are so terribly disinhibited and uncontrollable that contained classrooms are the only reasonable answer.

Some children need a self-contained setting but the school district has painfully few options within the district and can only offer to send the child on an hour bus ride to another school system.

We tend to take a step-wise course in implementing special services. Unless the child is severely impaired, we like to start with modifications within the regular class and add services as they become necessary. Stage I usually entails consulting with the teacher, making sure he or she is up to speed on ADHD and implementing classroom management programs tailored for mainstreamed settings. Stage II involves organizing more intensive services through the Resource Room program that may entail the child leaving class for an hour or more per day in order to receive individualized attention. (Some school districts are experimenting with "pull-in" programs that have the resource room teacher come into the classroom to provide special services.) Stage III options involve special class placement for most, if not all, of the child's day.

In our experience, most ADHD children require at least Stage II sorts of services in order to achieve satisfactorily. Regularly-scheduled opportunities for individualized attention can go a long way toward helping the ADHD child in school. Our bias is that Resource Room services are most helpful when they are primarily oriented toward review and organization of material rather than toward training of new skills using tasks unrelated to current classroom assignments. ADHD children often need, first and foremost, to sit down on a one-to-one basis and go over the assignments they had trouble focusing on in class or are simply unable to learn in a large-group setting. Sometimes the mere opportunity to spend a half hour at the end of the school day making sure, with the resource teacher, that all the homework assignments are understood and recorded has a whopping impact on an ADHD student's life.

A word about private versus public education for the ADHD child. Once again, we can only speak in generalities and you should not take our broad comments as necessarily relevant to your own situation. Many times parents will pull their child from the public school and enroll him in a parochial or private school with the expectation that the enhanced structure and smaller classes will make all the difference. Because private and parochial schools do indeed have smaller classes, there is greater opportunity for supervision and individual attention. We want to make it clear that we have seen this strategy produce the desired effects and allow a child to make considerable gains over what they were able to muster in the public setting. We also have to say, however, that the private school gambit has, more often than not, backfired. While private schools have smaller classes, they also have fewer options available by way of the range of teachers, support services, and learning environments. Many private schools just are not set up to handle children with special needs. They are more organized around higher achieving youngsters or, especially in certain religious schools, children who are unusually compliant. If a school is geared to manage special children, then it may represent a boon. If its investment is in working with only the Harvard-bound, watch out for a bust.

How Do You Know When More Intensive Services Are Required?

Although no tangible markers exist that can precisely determine when it is time to move to another stage of special services, there are signs that can point the way.

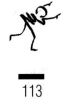

Certainly, when a child makes little if any progress academically over several months, it may well be that the current program does not allow for this child's learning. Unfortunately, some ADHD children are allowed to fail two and three years before there is movement toward appropriate services.

The decision becomes more obvious when the child's behavior deteriorates to the point that more time is spent in police actions than teaching. The flag signaling the need for a new course waves furiously when the school is reduced to managing a child's behavior primarily through exclusion. No amount of trips to the principal's office, thundering lectures, suspensions, or calls to a parent at work will make an ADHD child less ADHD if he is placed in a setting that does not meet his needs.

One thing that many parents, clinicians, and school officials do not appreciate is how frustrating it is for a teacher to deal with an ADHD child in an educational environment that in no way allows for the level of teaching necessary to help him learn. While it may often seem to parents that the teacher doesn't **want** to spend the time working with their child, it may well be that the setting simply does not afford the teacher the wherewithal to give the child what he needs. From the teacher's point of view, she's got 27 children in her class, all of whom warrant her attention, and then there's this one child who could easily be a full-time job all by himself. She's therefore torn between her responsibilities to the rest of the class and her full awareness that the ADHD student needs a disproportionate amount of her time if he is to achieve.

Sadly, some teachers deal with their frustrations by "taking it out on the child" and becoming angry with a situation that places demands on them that they cannot meet. The situation can cycle down to the point where the child becomes a "marked" man and is quickly excluded from class or even demeaned by the teacher in front of his peers. Other teachers are better able to know when it's time to rethink what is best for the child and, if necessary, pursue additional services. While any good teacher wants to feel that she can handle whatever is thrown at her, the best teachers have a keen sense when more is needed than they can offer. This sort of honesty and level-headedness best serves not only the ADHD child but also the rest of the class. An open-minded teacher can be a parent's best ally in knowing when additional services should be considered.

While we are wholeheartedly in favor of special services for ADHD children, we also want to warn you against gilding the treatment lily. We had one case in which the child was so heavily scheduled with resource room periods, occupational therapy, speech therapy, counseling and other services that he barely spent time in his classroom and actually missed critical instructional periods. The daily life of this highly disorganized youngster was spent in constant transition from one setting to another. Services have to be arranged sensibly in such a way that they are not themselves disruptive.

Parents need to be aware that the law requires children to be labeled as in need of special services before any such services can be implemented. As we mentioned earlier, the battles for ADHD children have usually been waged to secure labeling because the regulations fail to recognize ADHD as a handicapping condition. The labeling laws, however, are quintessential mixed blessings. On the one hand, labeling a child opens up a whole realm of possible services and legal recourse that would otherwise be unavailable. Once a child is identified under the law, the school is mandated to provide all necessary and appropriate services at its own expense. These services can range from a bus monitor to sit with a child, to psychotherapy, to residential treatment. At the same time, nobody (but especially a parent) likes to pin a label on a child that denotes disability or impairment. Parents also worry about a label being affixed to the school record and following the child even beyond the school years.

We urge parents to make judgments about labeling based on educational need and not on more vague concerns about the long-term impact of receiving special services. Parents need to accept that all options involve trade-offs and that their goal is to determine which option has most benefit to offer relative to the inherent risk. For example, placement in a special class undoubtedly can affect a child's self-esteem and social adjustment. But daily failure in a regular classroom which does not meet basic needs in any significant way can exact a heavy emotional toll as well. We had one child who, to the parents' astonishment, thanked them profusely for working with the school to place him in a special class. Despite his initial discomfort with going to the "Dummy" class, he soon found himself able to manage assignments and get adequate help when necessary. He told his parents, "I have a chance of doing things right in this class."

The decision to label a child is particularly onerous when the only option is "Emotionally Disturbed." Again, because there currently is no ADHD label and many ADHD children do not qualify as Learning Disabled, the ED designation is all that remains unless the school is willing to provide services informally (and some find ways of doing so). In those circumstances where it's the ED label or nothing, we encourage parents to look at the services offered more than at the label itself. We have children who are labeled ED but are essentially receiving a variety of resources nicely tailored to their ADHD needs. Also remember that there is an array of legal safeguards that are designed to protect confidentiality. Once the student is declassified, all information regarding the label must be expunged from his or her record.

What If The School Is Completely Uncooperative?

Many schools expend extraordinary effort to help children with special needs, even when budgets are tight and resources limited. We have seen teachers demonstrate remarkable dedication toward students, to the extent of risking their own jobs by fighting with administrators on a child's behalf. At the same time, we have been appalled at the stubbornness of some schools when faced with reasonable requests for special services. While we once thought that their unwillingness always stemmed from financial pressures, we have repeatedly been involved in situations in which it would have been much cheaper for the school to provide services than to fight the demand for them.

The law provides several means by which to challenge the school's decisions regarding your child, from meeting with the committee that oversees special educational services to calling a due process hearing which is presided over by an impartial judge. You can learn about these remedies by writing your state Education Department or by contacting your local learning disabilities association (the address for the national headquarters of the Learning Disabilities Association is listed at the end of this book).

If you are unsuccessful in securing services under regulations stemming from Public Law 94-142, another route open to you is a federal law called Section 504 of the Rehabilitation Act of 1973. The Office of Civil Rights within the Department of Education has ruled that ADHD/Hyperactive children are covered by the law if their condition substantially limits their ability to learn or to benefit from their educational program. You will find that, regardless of how it may sometimes seem, you have considerable legal clout and protection. If all calmer routes prove fruitless, you can also contact the Legal Services Administration which has an Educational Advocacy Branch. In our area, the lawyers and paralegal staff have been most effective in convincing schools to "do the right thing."

While you should know your rights and exercise them when necessary, it is clearly preferable that your relationship with the school stay on a cooperative, non-adversarial basis. It is not to your advantage to pursue more formal action until you are sure that all avenues for negotiation have been exhausted. Also remember that legal channels are time-consuming and that too many battles are won after the child's war has long been lost. You need to strike a fine balance between active cooperation with the school and energetic goading for changes you feel are warranted.

When you are confronted with a situation you consider unproductive or inappropriate for your child, you need to become a strenuous, forceful and informed presence at the school. This may entail that you make yourself more than a little bit of a nuisance or even that you band together with other parents to push for needed changes, especially if you find a profound lack of basic knowledge about ADHD/Hyperactivity.

We have met with parents whose advocacy efforts eventually led to extensive involvement on school boards and on special education committees. As one mother put it, "What it took was for me to become such a royal pain in the butt that they decided to provide the resource help just to keep me from driving them crazy." Believe it or not, we have also encountered families who have sold their homes in order to move to school districts with a more progressive attitude and range of educational options.

Schools often can be approached with a "You can pay me now or you can pay me later" argument for providing appropriate services. The ADHD child placed in an inappropriate setting will inevitably generate conflict and frustration that has to be dealt with in one fashion or another. The ADHD child who is underserved will require inordinate teacher involvement as well as intervention by the principal's office in response to misbehavior and noncompliance. "Wouldn't it be better to arrange for the resource room," we ask the principal, "than to spend your days dreaming up new ways of convincing Johnny to listen to the teacher and complete his assignments?"

Once again, your clinician should be of assistance in working with the school to develop a reasonable program. Sometimes a professional's statement on a fancy letterhead is all that it takes to convince a skeptical school official that your concerns are not those of an hysterical or overprotective parent.

We always tell parents to keep track of their contacts not only with school officials, but also with any other professionals involved in the child's comprehensive program. While it takes some discipline to maintain such a record, documentation of events can be a wonderful asset both in any legal actions as well as in making reliable historical reports when you are asked by a practitioner to review your child's life one more time with gusto. To help you get started with careful record keeping, we've put an "Agency Contact Log" and an "ADHD Events Log" at the end of this book.

What If Parents Are Uncooperative?

Several years ago, an imposing older gentleman stomped into our offices with a tape recorder under his arm and a burning desire for battle in his heart. He was livid because the school was intent on ruining his perfectly normal son, whom he referred to as his "seed," by suggesting that he be enrolled in a special classroom because of severe learning disabilities and attention deficits. Mr. Green went on at length about the evils of modern education and also played for us taped conversations with the school principal which he felt were clear evidence of conspiracy. He proclaimed his intention to fight against the school's recommendation until his dying day and left with his seed, wife and tape recorder in tow. To the school's absolute credit, they strenuously pursued special services for this boy at extreme expense of time and money. After negotiations with Mr. Green fell apart, they followed legal channels and eventually secured appropriate placement.

Parents resist services for about as many reasons as there are the proverbial fish in the sea. As we have discussed, parents often have a terrible time accepting the possibility that their child could be imperfect and require special assistance. It is easier for them to point to what they see as the educator's incompetence rather than their own child's vulnerabilities. Some parents are too brimming with guilt or beset with emotions that stem from personal or marital issues to look straightforwardly at the situation and arrive at reasonable conclusions. And other parents doggedly pursue services that aren't necessary or appropriate because of a nagging and unrealistic perception that their child is unusually needy of attention and protection.

As is so often the case, effective problem solving between parents and school breaks down quickly when communication is poor and both parties dash to extreme positions rather than to a common ground. In our experience, parents are likely to become most wary of a school's suggestions when they feel that the school hasn't performed a credible evaluation or when information has been conveyed in a way that is not understandable or meaningful.

A typical scenario involves the parent who calls us frantically in April because she just received a notice from the school that it is recommending the child be placed in a special class next year because of chronic academic difficulties. The parent, not having heard any negative reports from the teacher in months, is furious because she had made it clear early on that she wanted to be informed. She may then sign permission for an evaluation but never have the opportunity to sit down with the school psychologist to have the results explained. At the committee meeting she may be intimidated by the six or seven officials present and not understand or like the various terms being bandied about the table describing her son.

Let's say now that this mother has an unusually close relationship with this child because of her rocky marital history and his early medical problems. It doesn't take long before discussions about the child's education become tense and the parent balks at what may well be reasonable and appropriate suggestions. We have frequently found ourselves being called into these kinds of situations as a third party in order to help parents and school to better communicate their concerns and reach a resolution.

PRINCIPLE 19

There's Nothin' Better Than a Good Teacher

Finding a creative and competent teacher is often the most critical step in developing an educational program that works. Resource room assistance or classroom management programs are only as good as the people implementing them. You will find good teachers and bad teachers, teachers who may be good for some children but bad for yours, and teachers who are so talented and caring that there is surely a special place reserved for them in heaven.

It's this last sort of teacher that you must try to secure for your child because so many of his or her needs, if nothing else, call for a high level of teacher competence, dedication and ingenuity. This is particularly the case because there is no single educational technique for improving attention and achievement in ADHD/ Hyperactive children. What's needed is a teacher who can develop a range of interventions, figure out which work, and stick with the successful ones. Our first bit of advice to parents, especially during the springtime when plans are being laid for the following school year, is to call neighbors, talk to the principal, visit the school and do whatever it takes to find out who's the best teacher at the next grade level. Once you've located your best hope, then set about making sure that your child is enrolled in his or her class.

What Are Qualities of the Ideal Teacher for an ADHD Child?

The perfect teacher for an ADHD child need not be graced with magical powers or bear an uncanny resemblance to Mary Poppins or Mother Teresa. The essential requirements are that she (for the sake of balance and accurate reflection of reality we'll use the female gender) have solid teaching skills, a consistent dedication to her students, flexibility, and more than a bit of ingenuity. While there are some special techniques that may be helpful in teaching ADHD children, most strategies are simply founded upon good, solid teaching abilities.

As you will also hear in regard to parenting, the only real differences between teaching an ADHD and non-ADHD child is the degree to which you have room to deviate from excellence. With your other students, you can usually get away with being less clear in your instructions or occasionally disorganized in your management of the classroom. The roof won't fall in if you forget to deliver consistent consequences or redirection to task. ADHD children cut down on your room for error. Minor breakdowns in your own discipline as a teacher can lead to trying times.

Here's a list of some characteristics of our mythical Ideal Teacher. Again, the first item aside, you will probably say, "You're just talking about good teaching" — and you'll be right:

The Ideal Teacher (and Parent) for an ADHD Child

1. Thoroughly knowledgeable about ADHD/Hyperactivity and accepts the legitimacy of the disorder

2. Tough as nails about rules but always calm and positive

3. Ingenious about modifying teaching strategies and materials in order to match child's learning style

4. Tailors academic material to suit child's abilities and skills

5. Creates assignments that require as much activity on child's part as possible — Hates dittos and endless seatwork

6. Mixes high and low interest tasks in tune with child's predilections

7. Isn't into homework in a major way

8. Knows to back off when student's level of frustration begins to peak

9. Knows to back off when teacher's level of frustration begins to peak

10. Speaks clearly in brief, understandable sentences

11. Looks the child straight in the eye when communicating

12. Runs an absolutely predictable and organized classroom

13. Controls the classroom without being controlling

14. Provides immediate and consistent feedback (consequences) regarding behavior

15. Develops a private signal system with child to gently notify him when he's off task or acting inappropriately

16. Maintains close physical proximity without being intrusive

17. Ignores minor disruptions — Knows how to choose battles

18. Has no problem acting as an "Auxiliary Organizer" when appropriate and necessary — Makes sure child is organized for homework, parents are notified about school events, etc.

19. Maintains interest in the child as a person with interests, fears, and joys — even after a trying day

20. More than willing to call or meet with parents frequently to keep in step with other efforts

21. Has a sense of humor you wouldn't believe

So much of what we look for in teachers for ADHD children is a willingness to adapt to the child's handicap by experimenting with alternative methods of instruction. If a child learns math facts best in a game format, then our Ideal Teacher comes up with all sorts of intriguing math games. If the student completes the most work while seated under his desk or standing on his head, then she allows this to happen (but edges the student gradually toward more normal work habits). If the student produces the most if assignments are broken down into 10-minute instead of 20-minute segments, then the Ideal Teacher arranges the schedule accordingly. She knows that there's a firm distinction between structure and rigidity. A teacher can be flexible in her willingness to develop individualized programs but highly structured in the manner in which they are deployed.

The Ideal Teacher knows that, like it or not, she needs to spend extra time throughout the day helping the ADHD child keep organized. She may have to tape a checklist of assignments on his desk or inspect his backpack right before he leaves to make sure all the materials needed for homework are included. Even though the student should take full responsibility for personal organization, the Ideal Teacher knows that there are inherent limitations in the ADHD child's organizational abilities which dictate frequent compensations.

At the forefront of the teacher's mind are ideas about increasing the child's level of academic productivity and social adjustment. Of less consequence is concern about whether or not modifications instituted for the ADHD child are somehow unfair to the other students. So often we hear teachers say, "Your recommendations make sense, but it just wouldn't be right to let one child get away with fewer demands while the rest of the class has to meet the higher standards."

We try to convince these teachers that **fairness isn't when everyone gets the same, but when everyone gets what he needs.** Just as you wouldn't ask a blind child to copy class notes from the blackboard, you shouldn't ask a child incapable of sitting for more than 10 minutes to complete 30-minute assignments. It simply doesn't make sense. If anything, it would likely be a valuable lesson for other students to learn that individuals have unique needs and that we all have the responsibility to help as best we can in addressing them. If a class can deal sensitively with the notion of compensating for special needs, then all involved will benefit.

Doesn't the Special Attention Embarrass the ADHD Student and Isolate Him from His Peers?

Parents and teachers often worry that any sort of modifications to the child's program will set him apart from his peers to such an extent that he'll be marked as "different" and suffer the consequences. This is not an unfounded concern because children, as a group, have never been noted for undue tenderness and compassion in their dealings with classmates. It's also true that the

ADHD child is often of mixed minds about receiving special help. Upon minor amounts of reflection he may understand the need for modifications, but he also wants to be like others as much as possible.

While there may well be social side effects from any special treatment, they are rarely so serious as to justify doing nothing. To begin with, much of the goal in working with ADHD children is to help them adjust to their disability. They need to become comfortable with being a bit different and with needing modifications to their lifestyle that are aimed at helping them adjust. More than anything else, the ADHD child needs reassurance that he's neither crazy nor stupid. As we just mentioned, the teacher can do much to direct the class toward understanding of this problem and the rationale for special services or changes in expectations. Too frequently these sorts of issues are danced around or left without resolution.

The other thing to point out is that an ADHD child who does not get the extra help will tend to act in ways that are at least as alienating to peers. It may be "different" for a child to be the only one in the class on a behavior modification program, but it certainly sets a student apart when he is the only one who didn't finish his assignments or who was sent to the principal's office for inappropriate language. You can't deny modifications because of potential social repercussions. Those consequences will surface one way or another and, if handled properly, can take a productive course.

PRINCIPLE 20

Try To Work It Out So That the Child Wins — Or At Least Has More Than a Snowball's Chance

Underlying many of our suggestions about good teaching and parenting strategies is a plea for common sense. Nine year old Tammy's teacher described the behavior management program she's been using in her classroom over the past two months. "It just doesn't work," she told us, "Tammy doesn't respond at all." When asked to describe the program, she told us that Tammy had to have three weeks of perfect behavior in order to win an ice cream cone. "What's the longest Tammy has ever been able to maintain perfect behavior?," we asked. "Oh, maybe a day or two at best," came the response. "What are the chances she could string three perfect weeks together?" "Not great," the teacher told us.

All intervention strategies have to be designed in such a way that the child has a decent chance at success. We want the youngster to know from the outset that we are asking him to do things that are within his powers to attain. The moment a child senses that there's little chance of winning, all is lost. You can design the prettiest stickers and wax eloquently about the joys of adherence to the program, but always make sure that your expectations and goals are reasonable. In the case of Tammy, we had already heard her assessment of the teacher's program, "She's crazy if she thinks I could be good for three weeks. Forget that. And besides, I don't even like ice cream!"

Frustrations swirl around an ADHD child like sand in a windstorm. If the child isn't frustrated by demands for attention, then the teacher is frustrated by his unwillingness to tackle material. If the teacher isn't frustrated about the student's lack of productivity, then parents are frustrated because he doesn't seem to make progress.

Frustrations often spring from expectations gone awry. If you harbor the expectation that an ADHD child will function consistently over time, you will inevitably become frustrated when the ADHD roller coaster rises and falls. If your expectation is that all children must perform seatwork for 40 minutes every morning, everyone will become agitated when the extremely active six-year old barely makes it through 10 minutes. **Reasonable expectations make for happier campers.** More on this later.

A general who deploys his troops along too many fronts is vulnerable to stretching resources thin and thus leaving himself open to failure. An effective general always chooses his battles wisely. The same principle applies to effective management of the ADHD child. **Choose your battles!** If you attack all the problems at once, you'll frustrate yourself and the child. Before you know it, you'll wallow in a sea of charts, tokens, and rules. You'll generally be far better off sitting down with a piece of paper and listing two or three target problems that will be the starting point of your current efforts. Do your best to hold off focusing heavily on the million and one other issues that need attention but will have to wait in line. Once you get a handle on a few problems, you can always move on to others.

Much of our consultation to schools is aimed at helping them make reasonable decisions about which problems to attack and which to save for another day. It often seems like the story of the man who went to his doctor because he felt pain every time he raised his arm over his head and twirled it around. The doctor ran a series of tests over many weeks and eventually arrived at the diagnosis of an exotic form of arthritis. "So what's the treatment?," the patient asks. "Don't raise your arm over your head and twirl it around," comes the reply. This occasionally is the best approach to dealing with the ADHD child.

Because you can't solve all problems at once (and there may be a few that are, at least in the near term, insolvable), working around some of them is often the most prudent course. If ADHD Johnny will inevitably run afoul of the rules if left to walk to Art Class at the end of the line, then hold onto his hand while you walk with him at the front of the line. If he cannot yet tolerate riding on the school bus because he hangs out the window or starts fights, arrange for a bus monitor to sit with him or a smaller van for transportation. If you're not yet ready to deal with his inability to comply with demands in the gym class, then make special arrangements for his physical education. Knowing when to hold them, fold them, walk away, and run is as important a skill in managing ADHD children as it is in poker (at least according to the song).

PRINCIPLE 21

Dealing With the ADHD Child As a Little Criminal Will Get You Nowhere

Most ADHD children are remarkably adept at pressing all the wrong buttons on a daily basis. As a group, they are constantly trying the patience of teachers and parents. "It's like a storm that only lets up for a few minutes a day," one teacher reported. "Hardly an hour passes when I don't have to deal with something Jerry's said or done." Some teachers, but particularly those who don't understand ADHD, enter into a negative spiral which goes nowhere but down. They begin to view the ADHD child's impulsiveness and inattention as acts of will and defects of character rather than as symptoms of a handicap. Nobody wins.

If you're at the point where equilibrium is lost and you can't deal calmly with the child, it's time to take a step back (or toward the teacher's room) and get yourself on track. The last thing you want to do is become punitive and reactive to the ADHD student's behavior. If they can't leave school with much skill in English Composition, they should at least have a healthy self-image tucked under their arm. It's just an act of honesty and professionalism to acknowledge your limitations in dealing with a particular child and arrive at an alternative plan. You may take the upset as a cue that additional services are in order, or you might even feel it wise to throw in the towel and push for a change of teachers. What you don't want to become is more the problem than the cure by falling into a contest of wills.

PRINCIPLE 22

Homework — Beware the Law Of Diminishing Returns

While we've covered many suggestions regarding the education of ADHD children, there are a few pet peeves we haven't had a chance to harp on yet. One of our most enduring criticisms of the way some teachers deal with ADHD children concerns what we see as an overemphasis on homework. It is too common for parents of these youngsters to report on homework wars that can last two or three hours every night of the week! True, the rest of the children may get all the work completed in half or quarter the time, but that's why they're not diagnosed as ADHD.

Why make children who struggle through a whole day of demands for attention come home to several additional hours of drudgery? Too many children and parents can get worn down by the process and end up with completed homework but depleted energies. After a while, the ADHD child begins to see home and parents as another extension of school and teachers. Many opportunities for parents and child to enjoy each other and engage in mutually pleasurable activities are lost in the pursuit of completed assignments. This process wears everyone down and prevents children from learning that there's more to life than academic excellence.

More often than not, homework is rehearsal of material covered during the course of the day. While review is certainly helpful in reinforcing class lessons, there's a point of diminishing returns that appears quickly on the ADHD child's horizon. We ask teachers to assign no more than 30-45 minutes of homework for ADHD children in the elementary grades, and no more than an hour or so for older children. If an assignment entails completion of a project (such as a book report or science experiment), we encourage teachers to let parents know when the project is due and to schedule "check-in" points along the way so that progress can be monitored. This is to avoid the "Night Before" panic that can send households reeling. To the extent possible, it's best if complicated material and reports can be handled in school, perhaps during resource time.

Homework can also be an opportunity to finish work that the child failed to complete during school hours. In fact, some teachers end up sending enormous amounts of work home because they have been unable to get the child to do anything productive during the day. A parent should not be placed in the position of compensating for unsuccessful educational efforts. It is much more reasonable for the school to take responsibility for implementing strategies that will increase a child's work productivity.

While we have a problem when too much homework is assigned, we aren't suggesting that an ADHD child should never have the experience of dealing with this aspect of school. We just hate to see it get out of hand.

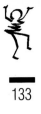

PRINCIPLE 23

Down With Education by Ditto

We don't know if it's our imaginations or not, but it seems to us that teachers are making increasingly heavy use of worksheets as a mainstay of educational efforts. We visited one classroom where the day essentially consisted of completing one mimeographed sheet after the next, with occasional "specials" (art, music, and gym) interspersed. The boy we were working with simply could not handle this pedagogical approach for more than 10 minutes at a time. After it became clear that his teacher was unwilling to modify her lesson plans, we prevailed upon the principal to switch the student to a teacher who had a more engaging method. The changes in the boy's productivity and mood were dramatic, so much so that tentative plans to place him on medication were shelved. As he put it, "I thought that if I had to do one more of Mrs. Brown's worksheets, my head would split open and dittos would come out. Mrs. Jones makes it interesting for me by making games out of the lessons and by not forcing me to do so much seatwork."

Just to reiterate one more time with gusto, ADHD children need material presented to them so that it captures their attention and breaks through the "thick barrier." The more captivating the material, the more likely that an ADHD student will pay attention and stick with the task. This is why computerized educational programs can be so successful with this group of children. It's a lot more interesting to learn spelling words in the course of helping a wizard find his way through an enchanted cave, than by means of mimeographed lists to be memorized. Similarly, the ADHD student is more likely to learn math facts as part of a game in which he has to save the world from nuclear annihilation, than by completing a series of worksheets. Never forget that ADHD children learn best when information is presented in digestible chunks of enticing material. The most successful teachers of ADHD children have an innate feel both for breaking up the lesson in manageable segments and for discovering ways of making it all fun.

PRINCIPLE 24

Increase Classroom Structure Any Which Way You Can

Having made global comments, we can now move on to other suggestions and specific techniques. Most of what we will discuss falls under the heading of "Structure, structure and more structure." As Dr. Barkley puts it, ADHD children require a prosthetic environment which, at every turn, enhances the amount of compensatory limits and consequences. ADHD children need structure the way a deaf child needs sign language. The ensuing discussions essentially detail ways of increasing the intensity and pervasiveness of structure and making sure that it follows the ADHD child at every turn.

What Would a Classroom Look Like in ADHD Heaven?

As we discussed earlier, children require different classroom settings depending on a host of factors such as age, problem severity, and intellectual ability. From our point of view, there is no one perfect classroom for every ADHD child. Nonetheless, we thought it would be worthwhile to speculate on the makeup of an Ideal Classroom for our Ideal Teacher. Let's assume that this classroom is for a relatively impaired seven year old ADHD boy who, by all accounts, cannot tolerate a regular classroom:

The Ideal Classroom for an ADHD Child

1.   No more than eight children (preferably 5-6) not all of whom are ADHD (some may have learning disabilities, speech and language impairments or other behavior problems)

2.   One trained ADHD teacher

3.   One trained aide with another available as needed

4.   Four walls and one door

5.   Extensive soundproofing

6.   Windows placed above height of tallest child

7.   Lines on the floor creating traffic lanes through the classroom (and through the rest of school building)

8.   Walls relatively replete with posters outlining the rules and extolling the virtues of planning ahead, feeling good about oneself, and socializing. Nothing stimulating but not barren or sterile either

9.   Bathroom at back of classroom

10. Daily schedule in bold letters on the board

11. Desks not too close together yet positioned in such a way that teacher can maintain close proximity to each student

12. An attention trainer on every desk (we'll describe these shortly)

13. A jar of tokens on the teacher's desk and a menu of possible prizes on the wall

14. A time-out room connected to classroom

15. Computer for every child located in separate section of the class

16. Observation room with one-way mirror so children can be observed by parents, staff, and outside professionals without disrupting the class. Observation room could also double as a "1 to 1" area for special instructions

17. A common area where children and teachers can sit and discuss group issues and feelings

18. Incandescent lighting and additive-free lunches (just kidding!)

Our Ideal Classroom, as you might imagine, is designed to allow the teacher and aide to exert unusual amounts of structure and monitoring. Notice that we are looking for a room that's conservatively stimulating in decoration but by no means sterile or boring. ADHD children need an optimal level of stimulation to function best. Too little of interest and the ADHD child will fill the void by acting up. Too much of interest and he will often become overstimulated and wound up. The challenge with ADHD children is Goldilockesque in that you're always having to find the porridge that's just right, whether it be the amount of clutter to allow in the classroom or the number of out-of-class experiences to program into a day.

You will find yourself having to play with the best seating arrangements. The common assumption, typically well-founded, is that the ADHD child does best in the front of the room where the teacher can keep an eye on him and maintain close contact. Nonetheless, we have worked with some children who are most productive when placed nearer the back of the room where they can move around without disrupting the classroom as much. One teacher told us, "If he's not right under my nose, it's much easier for me to ignore all the little annoyances that should be ignored. I just have to make sure to walk over to him often and keep him on track."

In general, the best classroom design allows for maximum teacher contact with a minimum of class disruption. This usually depends heavily on the teacher's style. We have watched many teachers who, unless they are over in a reading group, tend to stay close to their desk at the front of the room. With this teacher style, it may be important to keep a close eye on seating arrangements. Other teachers constantly roam about the classroom and never really park in one spot. They are often less focused on seating issues and more on finding ways to promote their mobility.

What Happens in Middle School with Team Teaching and Multiple Classrooms?

Parents and teachers have been known to break into a cold sweat when they contemplate their ADHD youngster moving into middle school or junior high where schedules involve more than one teacher and classroom. They wonder how a child who needs so much individual attention and structure can possibly survive constant changes in rooms and expectations. Such fears are often well-founded and prompt consideration of placement in contained classes or, at the least, of increased resource room involvement.

We have to say, though, that disaster hasn't struck as often as we have expected. Sometimes it even works out for the better for reasons about which we can only speculate. The shifts in classrooms during the day allow for sanctioned opportunities to move around the building. ADHD children often like knowing that every half hour or so they can get out of their chair and travel about the territory. A slate of teachers means that no single teacher must bear the brunt of the ADHD child's behavior for the full day. There's a bit of a tag-team phenomenon than can develop where a child is naturally passed on to a fresh individual just at the point when exasperation begins to crest.

Promotion to upper grades does, however, entail a far greater effort at coordination of services. The parent now has to communicate with five or six teachers instead of one. A heavier burden falls on the school's shoulders to integrate efforts and make sure that all teachers are maximizing structure and maintaining a reasonable degree of consistency in approach. Schools that are seriously invested in a team approach to each child find this level of coordination easier to manage. We have had most difficulty working with systems in which each teacher tends to act as an independent agent only loosely tied into a coherent program. Because the parent now has to connect with a multitude of teachers instead of one, schools need to help them have efficient communication with the team, perhaps through a coordinator or contact person who they know will work hard to integrate efforts.

Just because a child changes classes doesn't mean that all structure has to fall by the wayside. Assignments can be written in a special notebook (chained, of course, to a belt loop) and signed by each teacher at the end of class. Schedules can be adjusted to minimize the number of class changes and ensure that demanding courses are not timed one after the other. Study halls can be augmented with one-to-one time to check that the student is on schedule to complete long-term projects. In sum, an elementary school diploma does not signal an end to the need for creative structuring and horse sense.

Are There Classroom Management Programs Designed Especially for ADHD Children?

We literally have a closet full of programs designed for teaching ADHD children. They generally fall into one of two categories: Cognitive Behavior Modification (CBM) programs are designed to teach the child internal strategies for coping with situations requiring delay or self-control. They are based on the notion that ADHD children lack the ability to organize and regulate their behavior because, unlike their non-ADHD counterparts they fail to "stop, look, listen and think" before proceeding with a response to a situation. CBM advocates often speak about the problem ADHD children have "talking to themselves" in a way that allows for consideration of consequences, alternative coping strategies, and feedback. A CBM program tries to teach the ADHD child to think about the steps necessary to perform a task successfully. This sort of instruction is often delivered in special training sessions in which the therapist, using a game or activity such as checkers, models appropriate behavior and "thinks aloud" so the child can see how to handle a task in an organized manner.

While CBM makes good intuitive sense, research has generally failed to show consistent long-term benefits. The biggest problem concerns the issue of generalization: teaching a child a planning skill in one situation does not guarantee that it will transfer to another setting. As a matter a fact, generalization tends not to occur for most children. The exception may be when CBM techniques are woven into the fabric of the curriculum and of regular class activities. This application, though, requires that the teacher be fully trained in this program and organize her lessons with CBM as a guiding principle.

The other category of non-medical approaches involves systematically altering consequences for a child's behavior. This is based upon the notion that ADHD children require unusually clear-cut, consistent, and immediate consequences for their behavior. These "contingency management" programs are designed to create an environment for the child in which there are unusually clear rules, careful monitoring of behavior, and quick feedback. They are available both for the classroom and home. Some programs stress systematic, positive reinforcement of behavior by means of tokens, money or food. However, in the classroom these kinds of "token economies" are limited because interrupting a child while he or she is attending often leads to increased disruption. They also require considerable effort and discipline on the teacher's part. It's often hard for a teacher to dispense reinforcement on a consistent basis when so many other demands vie for his or her attention. An effective contingency management program also needs to be motivating and enriching for the child. Simply putting a child in a quiet space and dispensing poker chips rarely leads to improved attention and self-control.

It also turns out that children respond more favorably to the possibility of losing a reward than to the chances of winning one. In other words, children are more likely to comply with a command if they know they will lose a point (called "response cost") than if they simply earn a point for compliance (called "positive reward"). While some recoil at this notion because it sounds nasty, it actually translates more into a matter of phrasing than of substance. Under response cost principles you would say to the child, "Here are 10 chips you can have for the morning. Each one is worth 5 minutes on the computer games. If you don't break the rule about getting out of your seat, you get to keep all the chips. The only hitch is that I have to take one from you every time you break the rule."

The positive reward alternative just starts from the opposite side of the coin, "Every 10 minutes you sit in your seat I'm going to give you this chip which is worth 5 minutes of computer time." While some feel response cost approaches are punitive, we really don't think that this is so. Moreover, research indicates that it is the more effective strategy for dealing with classroom management.

A program that embodies the essential elements of effective contingency management was developed, along with our group, by Dr. Mark Rapport of the University of Hawaii. The Attention Training System (ATS) involves placing on the student's desk a small, electronic module with a counter and red light which the child knows as "Mr. Attention." The child is told that Mr. Attention will automatically award a point every minute that s/he pays attention to classroom assignments. At the end of the session, the child can convert earned points to minutes on the computer, extra time in the play area, or some other rewarding activity. However, if the child fails to attend to task, the teacher can, from anywhere in the room, press a button on a small module. Activation of this button causes a red light to shine on the student's module and a point to be deducted from the accumulated total. As such, the teacher can deliver systematic and immediate feedback without having to set timers or run across the room to dispense tokens or speak to the child.

Research on this technique, which incorporates both positive reward and response cost, indicates that it can be as effective as stimulant medication in increasing attention to academic activities. Equally important, the ATS approach sidesteps the issue of generalization because it operates during the course of normal classroom activities without special training sessions or participation in skill-building exercises that may not transfer. Schools that use the ATS report that it often allows children who would normally be moved to more contained settings to remain mainstreamed because the teacher can exert greater supervision without expending inordinate amounts of time and energy. Children like the ATS because reinforcement for good behavior is automatic and delivered by means of hi-tech gadgetry.

In the figures below you will find data from a study we conducted with six youngsters (three males and three females) between the ages of six and nine who participated in an after-school, psychoeducational treatment clinic for ADHD children. This weekly program was designed to increase a student's attentiveness and task persistence. In the figures, you will see the number of times that the child was coded as being off-task during each of the 13 sessions. Mr. Attention was not used during the first two or last two sessions so we could see the effect of this technique.

In five of the six cases, the children's level of attention improved from the two weeks of no treatment to the training phases, and then deteriorated once the ATS was removed. As such, the ATS appeared to provide structure sufficient to allow the child to improve the extent to which he or she maintained attention to school work. The one exception to the general pattern of improved on-task behavior was Subject 5, who showed initial improvement but then became inconsistent over the remaining weeks of the study. It is noteworthy that this youngster was eventually referred for residential treatment because of severe behavior problems and concerns about the possibility of manic-depressive illness.

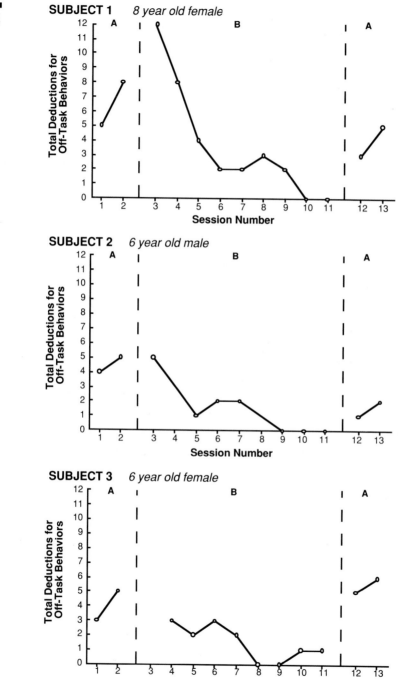

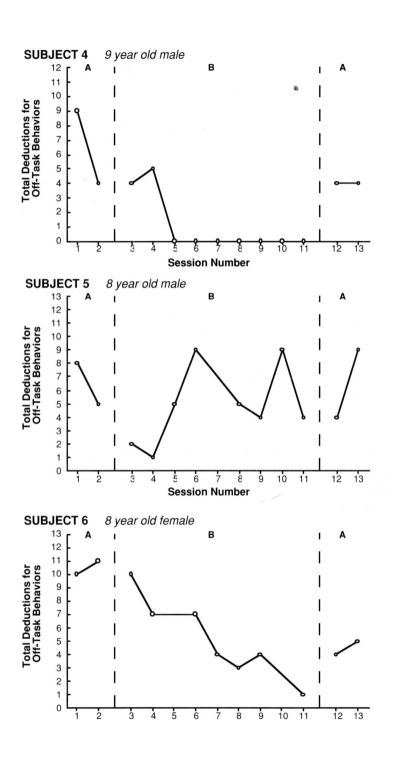

SUBJECT 4   *9 year old male*

SUBJECT 5   *8 year old male*

SUBJECT 6   *8 year old female*

While we are encouraged by the data being published on this technique, we are no more touting this system as the "ANSWER" any more than we did medication. There's an intriguing phenomenon that surrounds non-medical strategies: while there is not a grand program that cures all ills, seemingly minor interventions can make a world of difference. Daily checklists, token programs, frequent parent-teacher meetings, an assignment book, and other subtle changes in classroom management can produce noticeable improvements.

One last word before leaving our discussion of educational issues. While many schools are striving to incorporate effective programs for ADHD/Hyperactivity, we haven't yet heard of any that offer the level of service integration that would be ideal for treating ADHD children. In ADHD Heaven, the classroom program would be one piece of a total package that involved parent training, family therapy, and medication monitoring. Parents wouldn't need to go to the physician for medication issues, the psychologist for therapy, and the school for educational management. It would all be offered under one roof by a working team of professionals. So much wasted effort and so many missed opportunities could be avoided if there were not such splintering of services.

Being Asked To Participate in Your Child's Treatment Doesn't Mean You're To Blame

Our comments about parenting and home-based programs will be relatively brief because we have already covered the essential concepts in our discussion of educational management. The Ideal Parent isn't terribly different from the Ideal Teacher, and the Ideal Home isn't all that much unlike the Ideal Classroom. All basic principles underlying the schooling of an ADHD child hold true for the homestead: ever-present structure, consistency and immediacy of feedback over time and among adults, choosing battles, adapting the environment to compensate for disorganization and impulsiveness, and making sure that the child has a chance of winning.

Just like the teacher, you need to become an expert on ADHD/Hyperactivity, accept it as a legitimate disorder (and not punishment for sins committed during your misspent youth), find ways of helping your child adjust to his handicap, and avoid entering into the minefield of guilt and rage that always seems to loom for parents of ADHD children. Also like the educator, you have more than a few lesson plans to pursue every day. You need to teach your child to get himself ready for school in the morning, stand at the bus stop without decking all the neighbor children, complete homework assignments, eat a meal without having most of the food end up on the walls and floor, take the trash out after not the hundredth but the first request, visit Uncle Jim without blurting out how fat and weird he is, and get ready for bed in under three hours. Parents take an important step when they approach these issues in an educative mode that places a premium on level-headedness, effective problem solving, and humor.

While parent and teacher share similar mandates for dealing with the ADHD child, the parallels shouldn't be overdrawn. Yes, there's much for you to teach your child and your time is usually well-spent developing problem-solving strategies for managing the rough spots. But you're not just another teacher. Your relationship with your child can't be entirely oriented toward instruction and learning. You need to be viewed by your ADHD child as someone whose agenda is filled with activities and family experiences that sail well beyond the seas of education.

We make such a point of drawing the line between parent-as-teacher and parent-as-parent because it's so clear to us that raising an ADHD child can push mothers and fathers into emotional corners and family roles from which they can find it hard to escape. Parents have told us time and again how the child who drives them the craziest is also the one to whom they feel the closest. Perhaps it stems from the fact that children who are impulsive in their actions are also uninhibited in the expression of affection. Maybe it's because many ADHD children, even when in a helter-skelter of trouble, exude a certain innocence and naiveté which can be charming. Or it just might be that all the blood, sweat, and tears engendered by raising a child with special needs pulls emotional strings that normally are left unplucked. Whatever it is, parents can find it easy to get so caught up in "fixing the kid" that they forget to look beyond their role as teacher and case manager to their equally-important position as Mom and Dad.

How do our observations translate into actual suggestions? In many ways we'll be talking about in the next few pages. In part, we want to balance heavy directives about being structured, disciplined, consistent, and systematic in your child rearing with ones that also emphasize attention to emotions and family relationships. There's a certain point where you need to push the homework aside and snuggle up with your ADHD son on the sofa with a bowl of popcorn. Occasionally you just have to sit with your hands firmly clamped about your mouth and let him ramble on semi-incoherently about what happened at the baseball game, even though your impulse is to try to help him find the logic and language for his story. There will be days when you've got to stop issuing orders as well as correcting his every move, and let him just play and enjoy your quiet attentions. ADHD children require so much direction that it's sometimes hard to know when to back off and interact more as caring observer than as drill sergeant.

The number one pitfall of parenting an ADHD child is worrying so much about what the future might hold that you warp your handling of situations in the present. A mother with uncommon honesty told us about the train of thought that highballs through her brain every time her son Chris, who is all of six years old, runs afoul of a rule: "Let's say I find a fancy eraser in his pocket that I don't recognize and suspect he took impulsively off the desk of another student. Immediately I picture him following a life of crime because isn't stealing erasers just the first step behind shoplifting and car theft? And then I think to myself, 'How will this boy ever make it? He's just this side of suspension from kindergarten, he's a year behind in reading, and mothers in the neighborhood scatter when they see him coming down the street.' So now I have an antisocial, thieving school flunk-out on my hands who will be a burden on me and society for the rest of his days. I've got myself so worked up about what his taking of this eraser signifies for his future that I nearly bite his head off when he responds to my battle cries."

No one can blame the parent of a special child for being apprehensive about the future. Who doesn't want the best for his child and feel the pain of knowing that the road may be rocky? Nonetheless, it is critical for you to work at keeping the dread about the future from interfering with your parenting and, in particular, your reactions to events that are happening here and now.

The next trap to avoid is the "Cross to Bear" syndrome. If you have a child with ADHD, it might not take too long before your entire life begins to revolve around his needs. Hours are spent on the phone keeping in touch (or sometimes doing battle) with teachers, principals, and clinicians. You're always thinking about ways to overcome one obstacle or another in your child's path to normal adjustment. And before you know it, you get so caught up with his handicap that you lose perspective and leave little room for the rest of your life.

There's a special closeness that develops between a parent and a vulnerable child which brings a tear to the eye, but it can also go too far and stand in the way of healthy family life. Parents can become overly-resentful and intrusive when a child they work so hard to support engages in age-appropriate moves toward independence. They can also find it hard to let others intervene on a son or daughter's behalf because they've talked themselves into the notion that only they know what he needs.

When a parent becomes overly-tied to a child, nobody benefits. An overprotective parent is less likely to set firm and consistent limits because he or she walks on too many eggshells out of fear that the child can't tolerate demands for accountability or independence. Such a parent is also likely to set up the other parent as a villain from whom the child must be rescued. In an effort to maintain a close tie, the overprotective parent sometimes prevents others from establishing reasonable expectations and relationships with the child.

As we mentioned earlier, when parents are acting in ways that are counter-productive, the cloud of guilt is usually hovering nearby. Lurking in the minds of most parents of ADHD children is a reservoir of concern that somehow they are to blame for the child's condition and that others will discover their guilt. We've even had parents break down and cry when they talk about a family history of ADHD, because they feel guilty about passing down genetic traits.

When parents experience a high level of remorse, they tend to act in ways that make it difficult for others to help them. Some parents deal with guilt by refusing to take an active role in their child's treatment for fear that they will be judged culpable. They come to us and essentially say, "Here, fix the kid. We'll be back and pick him up after we get the dry cleaning." Parents worry that being asked to participate in treatment means that they are to blame. What they don't realize is that their involvement is crucial not because they are at fault, but because they are the ultimate keystone of any treatment program. They're the ones who have ultimate responsibility and can be most effective in implementing reasonable interventions. A parent's active participation is a clinician's best route to ensure effective treatment.

Anyone who works with ADHD children knows their capacity for making competent parents feel like fools.

You might have been voted National Mother of the Year but you still will spend more than a few hours shaking your head in bewilderment when trying to figure out how to deal with your ADHD child. Seeking help with child rearing should not be viewed as an admission of failure or incompetence but rather as an acknowledgement that some parent challenges are best handled with assistance.

You should always keep in mind another one of those elemental laws of human nature:

You Can't Help Others
Unless You First Help Yourself

While it's easy to adopt the role of selfless martyr and not look after your own mental and physical health, you should remember that a child's best ally is a reasonably stable and well-adjusted parent. It is not a crime against humanity for you to keep a close eye on your own state of mind and level of happiness. One of the best skills that a parent of special children can develop is the discipline to stay in touch with his or her own needs for rest, relaxation and joy.

How do you maintain your sanity? Schedule yourself mental health breaks throughout the week that allow you to get away from the family if only for a few minutes a day (but certainly for longer periods if at all possible). Take a walk, work on a hobby, exercise, go out to dinner without the children — find any ways that you can to remind yourself that you have a life of your own. On a regular basis, look to your spouse, parents, friends or babysitter to help you catch your breath. If no one can watch the children (perhaps because there's not a babysitter in the region your ADHD child hasn't terrorized), make it your business to create a chaos-free-zone in your house. A working lock on your bedroom door can at least allow for momentary respite.

One single mother we know instituted what she called the "Friday Night Video and Hot Bath" routine. Because there were no friends or family to spell her, she would cast her concerns about the impact of TV violence to the wind and rent the most engrossing videotaped movie she could find. She would set her three children and a box of favored cookies in front of the TV, let them know that they were not to leave the room except in case of fire or life-threatening injury, and she would then go upstairs for the cherished opportunity to take a steaming bath. Another mother made a habit of spending ten minutes every night watching her son sleep. A hellion awake, he apparently was angelic in an unconscious state. Seeing him in peaceful sleep somehow instilled in her a measure of calm and hopefulness.

One more point before we return to extolling the virtues of consistency and creative problem solving. It can be threatening to involve yourself in a treatment program if you're fearful about "other things" getting out. You might be hesitant, for example, to get involved in a parent training group because of a concern that weaknesses in your marriage will become apparent to others. It may be that you have your own unresolved issues about past failures or personal frustrations that are hard to ignore when you're sitting with a counselor talking about your underachieving child. It's always good practice to at least be aware of how your own marital and personal issues might interfere with your ability to be an effective parent and collaborator on a treatment team. It's even better practice to address such issues in therapy so that they will not diminish your capacity for coping.

PRINCIPLE 26

A Limit in Every Garage, a Consequence in Every Pot

By this point you know our penchant for focusing on structure and consistent feedback as guiding principles in establishing management programs for ADHD children. Many parents who come to see us have clearly lost control of their households; the child's victory is evident at every turn. Mom makes Chuck's bed because it's not worth fighting him to do it. His room is filled with toys because it was easier to give in to his in-store whinings than to say, "No!" The other children are generally at the mercy of his impulses and complain bitterly about their fate. Meanwhile Dad has volunteered for a position overseas as a way of avoiding the air of defeat that pervades the house.

Much of what needs to happen for the ADHD child at home is the gentle but effective restoration of parental authority. We don't mean that we outfit parents with six-shooters and handcuffs. We're talking about helping parents become more proactive and less reactive to the child's behavior. Random screaming and yelling are ineffective approaches for dealing with ADHD children. Beatings don't do much good either. (This point was driven home by an exasperated father who said, "I'm convinced I could rip his arm off and hit him over the head with it and there'd be no change in his behavior.")

What can help change a child's behavior is a home environment that is programmed to present clear-cut consequences to behavior and unwavering predictability of parental response. We want parents to have at their disposal a prearranged system for handling misbehavior rather than simply to react to problem situations with unique or arbitrary punishments.

A host of books offer detailed descriptions of child management strategies, and nearly all the titles listed in the "Resources" section have material on this subject. They provide tips for how to deal with a range of non-compliant behavior, including tantrums in public places, homework skirmishes, sibling conflicts, and chores. Parents have told us that the written material is quite useful in getting them thinking about ways to both compensate for their child's problems and to come up with predetermined strategies for dealing with noncompliance.

We have also heard that there are limitations to just reading about home management programs in books without professional guidance in applying the strategies to a family's special circumstances. For this reason, training programs have been developed to work directly with parents and children on these issues. One of the most popular was written by Dr. Barkley. The "Defiant Children" program lasts approximately twelve sessions and covers the full gamut of behavior management options in dealing with ADHD children. (There are even homework assignments for parents to complete each week.) Other programs, while somewhat different in presentation and emphasis, generally stress similar strategies.

At the heart of many of these programs are methods of providing the child with manageable rules and powerful incentives for compliance. Unfortunately, parents read about rewards and incentives for their children and, all too often, arch their back and declare, "I'm not going to bribe my kid to behave." Most of us prefer to think that children should do their homework and help around

the house out of a sense of responsibility and apprecia-
tion for the extensive parental sacrifices we have made
(as in, "After all I've done for you this weekend, the least
you could do for me is wash the car"). Most parents
would rather appeal to the child's altruism and love of
knowledge than get down to providing meaningful and
straightforward incentives for compliance.

While there are children who can be managed by
guilt and that famous phrase, "If you won't do it for me,
then at least do it for yourself," our ADHD patients never
fall into that category. You could lecture for days on the
value of a good education and the benefits of listening to
authority, yet not improve their performance even a little
bit. Patiently tell him that, in line with your agreement
with him, he'll lose 10 out of his 30 daily minutes of Nintendo (the unadulterated cocaine of childhood) if he
doesn't clean his room immediately, and you'll more
likely see a full laundry bag and the top of his desk.

While one can argue whether all children generally
do best with incentives (as opposed to less tangible rewards and punishments), no doubt exists for ADHD children. They need concrete consequences that have clear
value to them. Rewards need not be monetary. We have
seen children suddenly comply with rules for no other
reason than that they could earn minutes of TV time,
hours of baseball tossing with Dad, or Teenage Mutant
Ninja Turtle stickers. Children like tangible rules and
consequences; they are far more apt to respond favorably to your requests when the payoff is predictable.

These incentives are not bribes! Never forget that
bribery is when you pay somebody to perform an illegal
act. We would assume that nothing you are asking your
child to do falls under that heading. If it's bribery to pay
a child a dime for every morning that he is all ready

when the bus arrives, then it was bribery to pay the printer to have this book ready by the deadline. While there are most definitely reasons beyond receipt of reward or avoidance of punishment for listening to your parents, none are quite so compelling to the ADHD child.

We just want to remind you about a few basic principles of setting up reward and punishment systems for children. First off, stay away from all-or-nothing rewards, because once the child loses the opportunity to buy the prize or go to Burger King, all incentive for compliance is lost. We prefer rewards that can be graduated, such as money, time in a favorite activity, small candies, or cards and stickers. In this way, the child always has a chance at some reward, even after a bad day.

The response-cost approach to programming we mentioned previously is also applicable for home use. One clever parent, after hearing our description of the Mr. Attention program as a model for effective intervention, came back two weeks later wearing a broad smile. "We finally figured out how to get him to stop swearing in the house," she told us. "We put two dollars worth of nickels in a jar and told him that it would all be his by the end of the week. We also explained that we would have to take a nickel out every time we heard him swear. He tested us for two days to see if we were serious (we were), and that was the end of the gutter language." Not all families experience this degree of success, but clever development of strategies can bring good results.

Never stretch out payment of the reward beyond a meaningful period. Most 8 or 9 year-olds can tolerate weekly payoffs, but some need it on a daily basis. Also, remember that the best rewards are those that are chosen with the child's input. You might be surprised by some of the things children want to work for (our favorite was the boy who would set the table every night for the privilege of sitting at the "head" of a round table). As always, you need to experiment with a variety of strategies and discover what works. You also need to sit down regularly with your child and make appropriate modifications of rules and consequences.

Some families are able, without outside assistance, to sit down and negotiate a list of limits and consequences that are mutually agreeable and manageable for all involved. The list goes up on the refrigerator door, a jar of tokens appears on the counter, and the march begins. Many parents, however, find it a profitable use of professional help to secure advice on the efficient development of a home management program. An expert on structured programs can help you to avoid reinventing wheels and taking wrong turns. As we mentioned earlier, a competent professional involved in your case can also act as advocate, confessor, consultant, and therapist.

Regardless of how you come up with a behavior management program, stick with it! We have found that it's usually harder for parents to discipline themselves to stay with the program than it is for children. Parents need to support each other and maintain consistency in their enforcement of the rules. All of this is, needless to say, much easier said than done, but the extent to which parents work together and follow through on their program will directly affect outcome.

Don't Panic When You Find That Hyperactive Birds of a Feather Flock Together

It can be heart-wrenching to witness first hand the impact of the ADHD child's impulsiveness and overactivity on his relationships with peers. While some ADHD/Hyperactive youngsters experience success with peers, many are unlikely candidates for nominations to the post of "Most Popular" in the classroom or neighborhood. Their tendencies toward negative verbal interactions, bossiness, rule breaking, emotional outbursts and physical aggressiveness increase the chances that peers will reject them. Not renowned for patience in handling frustration, the ADHD child is all the more likely to deal with the lack of social acceptance by becoming even more unhappy and angry. Because a child's self-esteem is so dependent on a feeling of acceptance by peers, the ADHD child's vulnerability to social rejection represents another focus of concern for parents, teachers and mental health professionals.

Many parents wisely make a concerted effort to find opportunities in which their ADHD youngsters can experience acceptance by other children and learn social skills. Mothers and fathers are forever looking for an athletic activity, scouting organization, or religious youth group that might offer just the right setting for the ADHD child to develop a sense of belonging to a social network. Often parents become involved as a coach or den leader as a way of increasing the odds of success.

To the parents' frustration, ADHD children sometimes have an uncanny knack for hooking up with children who are themselves highly active and aggressive.
A child whose idea of a good time is to race blindfold-
ed down the street while perched on the handlebars of
his bicycle is not likely to seek out a friend who spends
hours patiently working on his stamp collection. Conversely, quiet children usually have trouble relating to
exuberant and active peers. Like their adult counterparts, friendships in childhood are often based upon
shared interests. For this reason, don't get your hopes
up too high that you will have much luck pairing
ADHD Andy with Silent Sam. As one mother told us, "I
used to think that if I just kept my rambunctious Billy
around his very mellow cousin long enough, then some
of the calm would rub off on my son. Instead, there
was just an unending series of conflicts between the
two boys, not to mention their mothers."

Our point here is that parents sometimes try to
overcompensate for their children's social difficulties by
loading the house with endless streams of "suitable"
children. While friendships can develop in this way, it
can also set up more opportunities for social failure.

We like to see parents engineer closely structured
and time-limited interactions with peers who might be
able to tolerate the ADHD child's active style. Initially,
you might want to have another child over to your
house for as little as a half hour and, without hovering,
structure the situation to minimize the possibility that
your ADHD child will lose control or interest. As always,
it's important to plan ahead, for example, by making
sure that your child knows the rules to games he might
play and that the other parent will be available should
the situation begin to deteriorate. If your youngster goes
over to a friend's house, you might let the other parent

know that you will be available at a moment's notice should your presence become necessary.

We also advise parents to think twice before planning all day treks, such as to the zoo or circus, with a retinue of friends. While these activities may be sufficiently intriguing and novel to maintain attention, they can also present too many opportunities in which misbehaviors are likely to occur. Again, you always want to place your child in situations in which there is a good likelihood of his coming out ahead.

When the ADHD child is with other youngsters, you may notice that he does a poor job of reading social cues and "saying the right things." Rather than jump on your child for rudeness, you may want to take a more educational approach and instruct him on what else he might have said or done in that situation. You can also practice social skills in a kind of game in which you rehearse the appropriate response in a given social setting. Remember that social graces are learned and, especially for ADHD children, not automatically incorporated into behavior.

We wish we could close this section with a simple formula for enhancing peer relationships for ADHD children but, unfortunately, this is one of the more vexing areas to manage. It's just hard to explain to a child with special needs why other children might not invite him to birthday parties or to their homes for sleepovers. Nobody will ever accuse children of being overly-kind to youngsters who are in some way different. Fortunately, a positive response to medication often entails improved social relationships, because the child's behavior is more acceptable to other children. In addition to a favorable drug response, we always hope that the child has (or develops) some special talent in realms, such as sports and music, that catch the eyes of his peers. ADHD children seem more tolerable to other children when they score the winning goal in soccer or perform masterfully at a gymnastics meet!

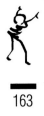

PRINCIPLE 28

Find (Or Organize) a Parent Support Group

One of the most encouraging developments over the past few years has been the emergence of a nationwide network of parent support groups. Having been associated with many of these organizations, we have been overwhelmed with the amount of effort and talent parents have invested in working with school systems to increase awareness of ADHD, sponsoring professional workshops, advocating with legislatures for changes in educational law, disseminating information to other parents, forming special summer camps for ADHD children, and providing a variety of other services to their communities.

These groups often start with a frustrated parent and a word processor, and then blossom into active and energetic forces to be reckoned with. The evidence of their effectiveness shines through in bright colors. The largest national group, called CH.A.D.D. (Children with Attention Deficit Disorder), has helped thousands of parents organize and has spearheaded a national effort to change the laws so that ADHD is included in the criteria for designating children as in need of special services. Local groups have won many victories in securing the cooperation of schools in providing programs tailored to the needs of ADHD youngsters.

Involvement in a support group offers several sources of benefit to parents. These groups serve as clearinghouses for information both formal (such as books, articles, and speakers) and informal (such as which pediatrician is most skilled in managing medication or where to find a clinician who understands classroom management). Because parents need to become educated before they can become effective, the parent support group provides a format for gaining knowledge efficiently.

There's also a group therapy component in these organizations that can sharply alter a parent's perceptions and diminish his sense of isolation. A mother told us, "Before going to the support group, I was convinced I was the only one in the world who had a child like Timmy. I found out pretty quickly that I wasn't the only one there who regularly plummeted into the depths of despair. It was good to be with people who understood what it's like to have an ADHD child." Parents often share suggestions and help each other through trying times. They also sponsor social events and special activities that draw together families who share a common experience. Another mother called us after she had attended a family picnic sponsored by one of the local associations. "It was wonderful to attend a function and know that my child wouldn't necessarily be the worst behaved!"

A parent support group can also be helpful to individual parents when conflict arises with a school, outside agency or clinician. In addition to providing information about your rights and names of others who can offer advice, your connection with an organization raises your status from that of a parent out in the wilderness to a member of an effective group of advocates. In this respect, your work with a parent group can return a high yield.

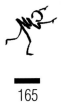

Hyperactive Children Who Succeeded Found an Adult Who Really Cared

When investigators study what happens to vulnerable or handicapped children upon reaching adulthood, one finding keeps resurfacing, regardless of the type of disability explored. If individuals who have succeeded are asked to look back and identify which factors they think contributed most to their positive outcome, they tell researchers about the impact of relationships they had with adults outside their family. They mention little league coaches who let them play despite their poor coordination, or scout leaders who were not put off by physical limitations, or a neighbor who would intervene when tempers ran high in the household.

The experience of being accepted and valued by someone other than your mother and father (who children figure have to love you whether they like you or not) seems to produce a protective coating around a child's self-esteem. Finding someone who knows your weaknesses but cares for you nonetheless is of inestimable value to all those children who might not always put their best foot forward.

We toyed with the idea of not relaying this bit of research data because there's not an awful lot a parent can do to connect a child with a caring adult. This may be one of those things you just hope upon hope comes along the way. But then we realized that people other than parents of ADHD children might read this passage and catch the message: children with special needs need special people to care.

PRINCIPLE 30

Keep Your Eyes on the Prize

We want to leave you with one last guiding principle about raising an ADHD child. It's easy to get so caught up in the battle to help our children achieve that we sometimes can go too far. We can forget how hard some of the youngsters have to struggle in order to make gains at school or home, and the extent to which many can be crushed beneath the pressures of educational demands. Some children we have known would have been better off with a somewhat lower reading level but a much higher self-esteem. For more severely impaired children, the daily battles can literally wear them out.

Ask yourself what it is that you want more than anything for your child. You might say that you want to see him go to college, or land a well-paying job, or become a successful businessperson. We all want to see our children achieve status and fame. But if you think about it, isn't what you hope for your child, more than anything else, that he or she end up as a reasonably happy and well-adjusted human being?

Years ago we saw two children within the space of three months, each of whom suffered from a combination of attention deficits and learning disabilities. Although different children in many ways, they were relatively similar in age (around 14 years), IQ (average), and in the severity of their problems (moderate). Terry was from a high-achieving family that was bound and determined that he graduate from high school with grades sufficiently respectable to allow for admission to college. They worked with Terry tirelessly every night and showed remarkable resourcefulness in finding the best special educational services and tutoring.

Steve's family took a different tack. They decided at an early stage that school was an experience they needed to help Steve survive rather than conquer, and invested much of their effort in propping up his self-esteem by helping him find other life activities that were rewarding. He became involved in scouting, baseball, and helping an uncle at a bike shop.

The two boys had sharply different outcomes, at least at this point ten years later. Terry graduated from high school intact but somewhat frayed and, at his parents' urgings, applied and was accepted to a small college. He passed his first semester, but only at considerable emotional cost in that he became morose and withdrawn. His parents were concerned about his lack of friends and uncharacteristically quick temper. By the end of the second semester his situation worsened as he became more depressed and uncommunicative. At the suggestion of the college counselor, he dropped out of school and returned to his family. Still encouraging him to pursue academic interests, the parents enrolled him in a local community college with the hope that a summer's rest would improve Terry's outlook.

Deterioration instead of improvement marked Terry's life over the next several years. He was chronically unhappy with himself and steadily became more angry. The last we heard, he is still living with his parents and, according to them, feels isolated and sad. They express no small amount of remorse at having pushed him so hard academically while overlooking his sense of well-being.

Steve made it through school with good independent living skills but a third-grade reading level. As a consequence of his involvement with scouting, he had developed an interest in woodworking. In his senior year he was in a work-study program that placed him in a company that refinishes furniture. The last we heard, Steve is happily employed by the same firm and, as best we can tell, enjoys his family life (he's married and has two little boys).

While there are many reasons why the two boys ended up at opposite poles of adjustment, we always felt that at least one factor had to do with the different amounts of pressure for achievement that each experienced during his early years. Terry achieved good grades but at a steep price, while Steve's grades, modest as they might have been, didn't become the sole focus of his existence. We are by no means advising that parents give up on expectations for academic achievement. It's just that children with these sorts of disabilities need to know that there's more to life than homework assignments and class grades.

Parents as a breed, but especially those with special children, always must search for balances. "How much do I push him to master Algebra and how much do I just help him to sneak by? Should I enroll her in ballet lessons even though she will have less time for homework or should I not push her on that front? Should I arrange for a tutor over the summer or should I let the poor kid be school-free for a few months? Do I really want to sign a contract for Karate or should I spare myself the expense and him another potential failure experience?" These sorts of questions forever taunt a parent (usually about 2 o'clock in the morning). While there are never easy answers to all the many questions, we generally feel that any error should be more on the side of ensuring a healthy self-esteem than on the sheer amount of academic material acquired.

ADHD children who succeed are not those who have achieved the highest grades or responded best to medication, but rather those who have found a comfortable niche in society. In the long run, the happy endings seem to follow stories of individuals who discovered a lifestyle that matched their strengths and skirted their weaknesses. A child who's at his best running about in the woods can make for a well-adjusted and content forest ranger. A gregarious, bouncy and charming ADHD boy can develop into the friendliest and most energetic salesperson in the territory (successful, too, if he has a well-organized secretary). While it's easy to fear the worst, remember that most ADHD children grow up to lead lives characterized by reasonable adjustment. From our vantage point, healthy adjustment isn't such a bad sight to set — and it's attainable, too.

In Closing . . . .

   While you are unquestionably entitled to moments of despair, we hope that, over time, you have found (or will gradually learn) ways of directing your energies toward active problem solving and adaptation. Parents who are well-adjusted to the trials and tribulations of raising an ADHD child seem to have accepted the inevitability of being firmly belted to a seat on the ADHD Roller Coaster. They don't see every bad day as a harbinger of total disaster or every good day as a sign that the problem is licked forever. Rather, they are happy for the good times but not overwrought when new challenges arise. Taking one day at a time is the best way of saving some sanity for another day. Good luck!

Resources

Books

Barkley, R.A. (1990). *Attention Deficit Hyperactivity Disorder: A handbook for diagnosis and treatment.* New York: Guilford Press.

Goldstein, S. & Goldstein, M. (1990). *Managing attention disorders in children: A guide for practitioners.* New York: Wiley & Sons.

Ingersoll, B. (1988). *Your hyperactive child: A parent's guide to coping with Attention Deficit Disorder.* New York: Doubleday. Order: Doubleday Readers Service, Dept. Z-46, PO Box 5071, Des Plaine, IL 60017-5071 (Hardcover $16.95; Paperback $7.95. Add $2.00 for shipping & handling).

Loney, J. (1987). *The young hyperactive child: Answers to questions about diagnosis, prognosis, and treatment.* New York: Haworth Press.

Parker, H. (1988). *The ADD Hyperactivity workbook for parents, teachers and kids.* Plantation, Florida: Impact Publications. Can be ordered for $12.95 plus $2.00 shipping per copy from: Impact Publications, Suite 102, 3000 Northwest 70th Avenue, Plantation, FL 33317.

Robin, A.L. & Foster, S.L. (1989). *Negotiating parent-adolescent conflict.* New York: Guilford Press.

Silver, L. (1984). *The misunderstood child: A guide for parents of LD children.* New York: McGraw Hill.

Turecki, S. & Tonner, L. (1985). *The difficult child.* New York: Bantam Books.

Wender, P.H. (1987). *The hyperactive child, adolescent, and adult: Attention Deficit Disorder through the life span.* New York: Oxford University Press.

Videotapes

Copeland, Edna D. (1989). *Understanding Attention Disorders.* 3 C's of Childhood, Inc. Orders: 3 C's of Childhood, P.O. Box 12389. Atlanta, GA 30355-2389.

Goldstein, S. & Goldstein, M. (1989). *Why won't my child pay attention.* Salt Lake City, UT: Neurology, Learning and Behavior Center. Orders: 670 East 3900 South, Suite 100, Salt Lake City, UT 84107, (801) 266 8895.

Goldstein, S. & Goldstein, M. (1990). *Educating inattentive children.* Salt Lake City, UT: Neurology, Learning and Behavior Center. Orders: 670 East 3900 South, Suite 100, Salt Lake City, UT 84107, (801) 266-8895.

Pamphlets

"Attention Deficit Disorders" written by Dr. Larry Silver and published by CIBA. Orders: CIBA Pharmaceuticals, 556 Morris Avenue, Summit, NJ 07901 Attn: Sales Services.

"ADHD Hyperactive Children" by Dr. A. Mervyn Fox from Children's Hospital in London, Ontario. Orders: Send $4 to cover printing and mailing costs to: Gordon Systems, Inc., PO Box 746, DeWitt, NY 13214.

"A Parent's Guide: Attention Deficit Disorders in Children" and a "Teacher's Guide: Attention Deficit Disorders in Children" are two pamphlets by Sam Goldstein and Michael Goldstein. Orders: The Neurology, Learning & Behavior Center, 670 East 3900 South, Suite 100, Salt Lake City, UT 84107, (801) 266-8895.

"Facts about Childhood Hyperactivity" by James Hadley is available from the federal government. Orders: NICHD, PO Box 29111, Washington, DC 20040

174

Training Programs

The Attention Training System (ATS) developed by Mark Rapport and Michael Gordon. Order: Gordon Systems, Inc., PO Box 746, DeWitt, NY 13214, (315) 446-4849. (This is also the address for inquiries regarding the Gordon Diagnostic System.)

Defiant Children: A Clinician's Manual for Parent Training by Russell A. Barkley. Order: The Guilford Press, 72 Spring Street, New York, NY 10012.

1-2-3 Magic by Thomas Phelan. Order:Thomas Phelan, Ph.D., 507 Thornhill Drive., Carol Stream, IL 60188.

National Organizations

Children with Attention Deficit Disorders (CH.A.D.D.)
1859 North Pine Island Road
Suite 185
Plantation, FL 33322
(305) 384-6869

Attention Deficit Disorders Association (A.D.D.A.)
8091 South Ireland Way
Aurora, CO 80016
(800) 487-2282

Learning Disabilities Association of America
4156 Library Road
Pittsburgh, PA 15234
(412) 341-1515

Agency Contact Log

Date	Phone or Meeting?	What Happened?	What Next?

Date	Phone or Meeting?	What Happened?	What Next?

ADHD Events Log

Date	What Happened?	Follow-Up?

Date	What Happened?	Follow-Up?